THE COMPLETE
Kid's
ALLERGY
AND
ASTHMA
GUIDE

THE COMPLETE
Kid's
ALLERGY
AND
ASTHMA
GUIDE

THE PARENT'S HANDBOOK
FOR CHILDREN OF ALL AGES

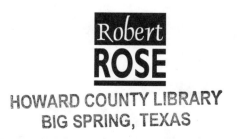

Robert
ROSE

National Library of Canada Cataloguing in Publication

The complete kid's allergy & asthma guide: allergy and asthma information for kids of all ages / general editor, Milton Gold.

Includes index.
ISBN 0-7788-0079-2 (bound).—ISBN 0-7788-0078-4 (pbk.)

1. Allergy in children—Popular works.
2. Asthma in children—Popular works.
I. Gold, Milton

RJ386.C64 2003   618.92'97   C2003-901472-X

Design & Production: PageWave Graphics Inc.
Editor: Fina Scroppo
Copy Editor/Proofreader: Ellen Rosenberg
Contributing Editor: Liza Finlay
Indexer: Barbara Schon
Illustrator: Gordon Sauvé/Three In A Box

We acknowledge the financial support of the Government of Canada through the Book Publishing Industry Development Program (BPIDP) for our publishing activities.

Published by Robert Rose Inc.
120 Eglinton Avenue East, Suite 800, Toronto, Canada M4P 1E2
Tel: (416) 322-6552 Fax: (416) 322-6936

Printed in Canada

1 2 3 4 5 6 7 GP 09 08 07 06 05 04 03

ACKNOWLEDGMENTS

THE GENERAL EDITOR AND ASSOCIATE EDITORS would like to thank the following people for their contributions. First, we'd like to thank the Hospital for Sick Children together with Robert Rose Inc. for giving us the opportunity to create such an important book. Thank you also to the various authors, for their hard work and dedication in creating individual chapters based on the most up-to-date research.

We'd also like to acknowledge Dr. Chaim Roifman, chief of the Division of Immunology/ Allergy at the Hospital for Sick Children, for his support of this project. To our publisher, Bob Dees, we thank him for his guidance and patience through this process, and to our editor, Fina Scroppo, we thank her for her accommodating approach, as well as thoughtful suggestions and patience, all of which allowed this book to reach its final stages. To Joseph Gisini and his design team at PageWave Graphics Inc., thanks for creating an easy-to-read format to help educate readers. And for their inspiration, we'd like to pay special tribute to the pioneers in the field of allergic diseases.

A special thanks goes to our families for their ongoing support throughout this process. We are grateful to the associate editors for their hard work and dedication in the production of this book. The associate editors, in turn, would like to especially thank Dr. Milton Gold for all his hard work and energy in ensuring this book was of the highest quality.

CONTENTS

INTRODUCTION

ABOUT ONE-QUARTER OF ALL CHILDREN SUFFER from some sort of allergic disorder, such as asthma, hay fever, food allergies or eczema. For a child, an allergy can be daunting and difficult to manage. For parents, a child's allergic condition can be confusing, frustrating and sometimes frightening.

The Complete Kid's Allergy and Asthma Guide is designed to give parents and caregivers comprehensive, authoritative information with common-sense guidelines, recommendations and tips on dealing with the asthmatic condition and the allergic problems that children can experience. Parents can rest assured they're reading about the most up-to-date, expert advice from allergy specialists at the world-renowned The Hospital for Sick Children.

While this book is only a starting point to helping you cope with your child's allergies, you can count on finding a wealth of useful information, including advances in diagnosing specific allergic conditions, how to minimize allergic reactions and how to avoid allergens and irritants. We understand how inundated you can be with all the 'news' about allergies, so we've provided an easy-to-read guide that will help to dispel some

common misconceptions and educate you on
the most appropriate care for your child's allergic
problems. This is truly a parent's handbook
you can share with friends, family and children
of all ages.

The book has been divided into four parts to
help you navigate more easily through the pages.
In Part 1, you'll get a summary of common allergic
conditions and allergic testing. Part 2 features
specifics on each allergic condition, while Part 3
will arm you with advice on dealing with allergies
and asthma. In Part 4, we've included the latest
research on the prevention of allergies. You'll also
find a useful glossary to help you cut through the
medical jargon and a listing of resources you can
continually tap into to stay current.

The information in this book has been compiled
using the latest research, current medical studies
and a wealth of experience the authors have gained
while treating childhood allergic conditions. Now,
all of this has been compiled in one volume and
passed onto you and your family. We hope you find
it valuable as we continue to make advances in
understanding and treating allergic conditions so
that allergic children and adults alike can live
healthy, normal lives.

CONTRIBUTORS

General Editor

Milton Gold, B.Sc., MD, FRCPC, FAAP, Diplomate
Am. Board of Allergy and Immunology
Associate Professor of Pediatrics, University of Toronto
Staff Physician, Division of Immunology/Allergy
The Hospital for Sick Children
Toronto, Canada

Associate Editors

Adelle R. Atkinson, MD, FRCPC, FAAP
Assistant Professor of Pediatrics, University of Toronto
Staff Physician, Division of Immunology/Allergy
Bone Marrow Transplant Medicine
The Hospital for Sick Children
Toronto, Canada

Sasson Lavi, MD, FRCPC, Diplomate Am. Board
of Pediatrics, Diplomate Am. Board of Allergy
and Immunology
Assistant Professor of Pediatrics, University of Toronto
Staff Physician, Division of Immunology/Allergy
The Hospital for Sick Children
Toronto, Canada

David Hummel, MB, ChB, FRCPC, Diplomate Am.
Board of Allergy and Immunology
Assistant Professor of Pediatrics, University of Toronto
Staff Physician, Division of Immunology/Allergy
The Hospital for Sick Children
Toronto, Canada

Other Contributors

Gordon Donsky, MD, FRCPC, FAAP
Assistant Professor of Pediatrics, University of Toronto
Senior Staff Physician, Division of Immunology/Allergy
The Hospital for Sick Children
Toronto, Canada

Suleiman Eisa, MBBS, FAAP, FRCPC
Clinical Fellow, Division of Immunology/Allergy
The Hospital for Sick Children
Toronto, Canada

Howard Langer, MD, FRCPC
Associate Professor of Pediatrics, University of Toronto
Staff Physician, Division of Immunology/Allergy
The Hospital for Sick Children
Toronto, Canada

Charlotte D'E. Miller, MD, FRCPC
Lecturer, Division of Respiratory Medicine
The Hospital for Sick Children
Toronto, Canada

Maria Triassi, MD, FRCPC, FAAP
Clinical Associate, Division of Immunology/Allergy
The Hospital for Sick Children
Toronto, Canada

Elisabeth White, RN, BScN, MS
Allergy Nurse Coordinator
Division of Immunology/Allergy
The Hospital for Sick Children
Toronto, Canada

Jane Salter, MD, FRCSC
Past President
Anaphylaxis Canada

PART 1

Introduction to Kid's Allergies & Asthma

Chapter

1

INTRODUCTION TO ALLERGIES

When Your Child Has An Allergy

ALLERGIC DISORDERS SUCH AS ASTHMA, HAY FEVER and eczema are some of the most common chronic health conditions among North Americans. For children, living with allergies can bring awful symptoms, from a simple stuffy nose to hives to difficulty breathing. Together, allergic disorders are responsible for many visits to the doctor's office and absenteeism from school. Many aspects of these disorders are still not fully understood and researchers around the world continue to study their causes, effects and methods of treatment. But we're making advances, helping children and adults with allergies live healthy, normal lives.

The Latest Buzzword

◆ ◆ ◆ ◆ ◆

Allergies are one of the most common health conditions and can cause a series of reactions, from a simple runny nose or rash, to more severe symptoms like having difficulty breathing, throat tightening and shock. Fortunately, allergies are rarely life-threatening.

Who's Affected?

5 FACTS THAT COULD AFFECT YOU

1. It's estimated that allergies affect 30 to 35 percent of the population, and that number keeps increasing, according to the latest research.

2. The most common allergic disease is allergic rhinitis (seasonal and year-round), with about 20 percent of individuals experiencing typical symptoms as a runny nose, sneezing and itchy, watery eyes.

3. One of the fastest growing diseases is asthma. It affects double the amount of children than adults.

4. Two to four percent of children experience food allergies, however, many of them will outgrow them before starting school.

5. Anaphylaxis, a severe allergic reaction to foods, medications or insect stings, affects one to two percent of North Americans.

How Does An Allergy Develop?

An allergy is the body's reaction to a substance (allergen) that does not generally produce harmful effects in the majority of people. You and your child can come into contact with allergens in several different environments and in a number of ways: by breathing, eating or drinking, touching, coming near or having them injected into your bodies.

? Did You Know...

In the last 20 years, allergic diseases such as asthma, food allergies and hay fever have increased significantly.

Common Allergens

The most common allergens in North America include:

Nonfood allergens	Food allergens
• Pollens (trees, grasses, weeds)	• Peanuts
• Molds	• Nuts
• House dust mites	• Shellfish
• Animal products such as dander (skin scales), saliva or urine	• Fish
	• Milk
• Drugs	• Eggs
• Latex	• Wheat
• Insects	• Soy
	• Sesame seeds

Your immune system produces different antibodies (proteins), such as IgG, IgA and IgM, to fight bacteria and viruses throughout your body. When you have allergies, your immune system overreacts and produces antibodies; those that react against allergens are called IgE. IgE antibodies bind and react on the surface of specialized cells called "mast cells," which are found on the lining of the nose, lungs, skin and intestines. Once the allergens come in contact with these cells, they release many chemicals, including histamine, which produce changes in various parts of the body, such as hives, swelling of the nose and chest linings and increased production of mucus. These changes are referred to as "inflammation" and cause a variety of symptoms. (See "Does Your Child Have An Allergic Problem?" right.)

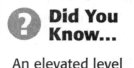 **Did You Know...**

An elevated level of IgE may suggest the presence of allergies.

Irritant Connection

People with allergies also tend to have an increased sensitivity to various "irritants," substances that do not normally cause an allergic reaction. These include:

• Cold air, damp weather

• Rapid changes in humidity or temperature

• Tobacco or fireplace smoke

• Strong odors or sprays

• Pollution

• Exercise

Does Your Child Have An Allergic Problem?

Every summer, five-year-old Michael has a stuffy, itchy nose. There's a clear watery fluid running from his nose and he's sneezing frequently. As a parent, you're often wondering: "Is he coming down with a cold or does he have an allergy?" This section will help you answer this question.

It's not always easy to determine whether your child has allergies. In fact, many of the same symptoms caused by allergies are also caused by other conditions. Before you start treating a child's allergy, consult your doctor. Here are some signs that might indicate an allergy:

✓ Always seems to have a cold

✓ Colds last longer than several weeks

✓ Runny, itchy or congested nose

✓ Frequent sneezing

✓ Mouth breathing, snoring, sniffling

✓ Coughing, wheezing; chest congestion

✓ Rapid or difficulty breathing

✓ Repeated nose bleeds

✓ Frequent throat clearing; itchy throat

✓ Headaches

✓ Frequent ear infections

✓ High arched palate, narrow chin, overbite

✓ Swollen, red or watery eyes; dark circles under eyes

✓ Eczematous-type skin rashes or hives

✓ Vomiting, diarrhea, abdominal cramping

✓ **FACT**

No I.D. Required

Allergies and asthma can occur at any age, but in most cases, they happen during childhood or early adulthood.

Colds Vs. Allergies

It can be difficult to tell the difference between your child's cold or allergies, especially in the early days of experiencing symptoms. Here are a few ways:

Symptom	Cold	Allergy
Mucus secretions	varies from clear and runny to yellowish and thick	clear and runny
Nose/eyes/throat/ears	no itch	itchy
Sneezing	sporadically	rapid sequence; usually around an allergen (e.g., dog, dust)
Duration of symptom	less than 2 weeks	more than 2 weeks

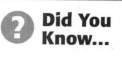

Did You Know...

What we commonly refer to as allergies is actually a number of allergic disorders, from asthma to hay fever to food allergies.

When Genes Matter

Some children are more likely to have allergic problems — in part because of strong hereditary links. If you have an allergic condition, such as asthma, hay fever, eczema or a food allergy, your child will also have a much higher chance of having an allergic problem. If only one parent has an allergy, the chances are between 30 percent and 50 percent. There's no certainty about the strength of allergies — children's allergies can be worse, milder or the same as their parents'. And, there is no set age at which these allergies can develop — they can appear during childhood, adolescence or in the adult years.

Family Connections

Research has shown that some allergic conditions seem to run in families. They include food allergies, allergies affecting the nose (allergic rhinitis, also known as hay fever), or chest (asthma), and sometimes the skin (eczema). Other allergic conditions that do not have such strong family relationships include hives, drug reactions, insect stings and latex reactions.

Strong Links

◆ ◆ ◆ ◆ ◆

If both you and your spouse have an allergic condition, your child's chances of having an allergic condition are between 50 and 70 percent. If you and your spouse have the **same** allergic problem, then your child's chances of having the same condition are about 80 percent.

Allergic Diseases

We tend to think of allergies as one disorder, but there are a number of conditions that are categorized as allergies, each with its own set of symptoms, diagnoses and treatment options. Each allergy will be discussed in more detail in the coming chapters — here's an overview of the main allergies that can affect your child.

ASTHMA

Symptoms
Patients with asthma are usually predisposed to having breathing problems when exposed to foreign substances. The most common symptom is wheezing, which is a high-pitched, whistling type of breathing, although wheezing doesn't always happen. It tends to be more pronounced on expiration (when breathing air out) rather than inspiration (breathing air in). Chest tightness, shortness of breath and a persistent cough accompany the wheezing. The cough is worse at night and may produce a thick yellow discharge.

Asthma Has No Face

◆ ◆ ◆ ◆ ◆

Asthma can begin at any age. The age of onset occurs most frequently during the first 10 years of life. It's more common in boys than girls by a ratio of 3:2.

Triggers

All these symptoms may be aggravated by physical activity, extreme weather (hot, humid and cold, dry), smog, allergens, fumes, tobacco smoke, strong odors, and even laughing. Episodes of wheezing tend to be more frequent during the winter months.

Measuring Sticks

A doctor will measure the severity of your child's asthma by noting the following:

• Days of school missed

• Night-time symptoms

• Ability to do physical activity

• Visits to the emergency department and hospital admissions

• Amount of medication used

• Pulmonary function tests (breathing tests to determine the degree of asthma)

Diagnosis

The physician will look for deformity of the chest and severity of wheezing when your child is being examined. Although a deformed chest was common among asthmatics during the 1960s and '70s, the introduction of inhaled corticosteroids has made it a rare physical finding. During a symptom-free period, the physician may ask your child to breathe out forcefully in order to bring out any wheezing (see "What Is Allergy Testing?" on page 32).

Is My Asthma Allergic?

The best way to determine an allergic connection is to keep an eye out for allergens. So, if your child is exposed to an allergen such as a cat, dog, dust, etc., there might be an allergic component to the asthma. If the wheezing tends to be seasonal, particularly from early spring until fall, the asthma may be related to pollen exposure. During the winter months, asthma may be associated with indoor allergens, such as, house dust mites, molds or animal danders. Allergy skin tests may help to confirm any offending allergens.

RHINITIS (Seasonal or Hay Fever, Non-seasonal and Year-round Allergies)

Symptoms

The most common symptoms of this condition are sneezing, itching, clear watery discharge and, eventually, a blocked nose. Less frequent symptoms include dull headaches, nosebleeds and excessive clearing of the throat. Your child may also complain of itchy ears, throat and palate. These symptoms occur within a few minutes after being exposed to an allergen, such as pollens (most commonly weeds, grasses, trees), animals (usually cats, dogs, horses) or other inhalants (house dust mites, molds, food products such as various flours). If the symptoms are seasonal, as in the case with hay fever, they're usually attributed to pollens and outdoor molds.

Triggers

Depending on the season, different triggers can prompt symptoms. Tree pollens are usually the cause in the spring, grass pollens in the summer, and ragweed in late summer and early fall. Outdoor molds tend to be a problem from early spring to late fall and during the winter months, indoor allergens, such as molds, house dust mites and animal danders, cause discomfort.

When the symptoms are seasonal or occur immediately after being exposed to other inhalants, for example, cat dander, the diagnosis is fairly simple. However, when the symptoms occur throughout the year, the condition is known as *perennial allergic rhinitis* or year-round allergies. Other conditions may have similar symptoms.

The common cold can often mimic allergic rhinitis. Although a cold's symptoms don't last throughout the year, they may linger for a few weeks, making it difficult for parents to treat a child's discomfort (for more information, see "Colds Vs. Allergies" earlier in this chapter). Other conditions such as adenoid swelling, nasal polyps, *rhinitis medicamentosa* (stuffy nose from overusing over-the-counter nasal sprays), and *vasomotor rhinitis* (drippy nose from changes in temperature or other irritants) may resemble allergic rhinitis. When no apparent cause is found for the nasal symptoms, the condition is known as *non-specific rhinitis*. Don't assume that any condition with nasal symptoms has an allergic basis — make an appointment with your child's doctor for appropriate testing.

Diagnosis

During an examination, your child's doctor will look for clear nasal discharge and swollen linings of the nostrils. If the nostrils are obstructed and, therefore, there's decreased airflow, your child will likely be breathing through his mouth.

Allergy skin tests help to confirm that an allergy, and sometimes a specific allergen, is causing symptoms (see "Who Can Be Tested?" on page 32). A positive result will be marked by a wheal or welt that is at least 3 mm in size. The most common

---

Scarce Signs

◆ ◆ ◆ ◆ ◆

Other less common signs that could suggest allergies are:

Allergic shiners — eyelids are a blueish colour because the veins in the lower eyelids, as well as the nose, are congested from a few days to weeks.

A **horizontal crease** across the lower part of the nose — this happens when a child repeatedly pushes the lower part of the nose upwards over a prolonged time.

allergens tested are pollens, house dust mites, animal danders and molds. If skin tests don't reveal an allergy, the child's physician may need to run other tests to rule out other causes of nasal problems.

Eye Allergies (Allergic Conjunctivitis)

The majority of patients with allergic rhinitis will also have eye symptoms. Sometimes they may occur without nasal symptoms, or if nasal symptoms are seasonal, eye symptoms will also be seasonal. Typical symptoms include swelling of the eyelids, burning and itchy eyes, and watery or mucus eye discharge. Occasionally, the sclera (the whites of the eyes) may become very swollen and look as if they were about to explode, even though you don't have to worry that this will really happen. This symptom is known as *chemosis* and rarely lasts more than a few hours.

Other allergic problems that can occur around the eye, particularly the eyelids include *angioedema* and *contact dermatitis*. Angioedema (or swelling) of the eyelid may occur as part of a generalized allergic reaction or as an isolated symptom. Contact dermatitis is a scaly, red rash that occurs a few hours or days following contact with an allergen around the eye. (See *Chapter 4: Skin Conditions*.)

SKIN CONDITIONS

Eczema (Atopic Dermatitis)

Symptoms

The majority of atopic dermatitis starts during the first five years of life. It's a chronic scaly red rash that usually begins on the cheeks. It can be an extremely itchy rash that leads to constant scratching and, eventually, cause bleeding from the affected areas. During the first year, it tends to spread to the creases — the elbows, knees, wrists, ears, neck and eyelids. After puberty, it commonly occurs on the hands, fingers and feet.

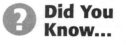

Did You Know...

Hives can be caused by factors with no allergic origin. For example, hives can be brought on by extremely cold temperatures or cold objects.

Triggers

Do food allergies cause atopic dermatitis? People with eczema have a higher incidence of food allergies, but the concept that they cause eczema is controversial. In a few patients, certain foods seem to aggravate eczema, and avoiding the food seems to improve the condition. However, up to 80 percent of individuals with eczema end up with other allergic diseases — either allergic rhinitis or asthma. At the present time, there is no evidence that atopic dermatitis is caused by an allergy.

Diagnosis

The physician will look at the nature of the rash, combined with your child's medical history. Skin testing may be conducted to look for allergies that could be aggravating a skin condition. Eczema can also be aggravated by heat and contact with rough surfaces, among other factors.

Other Skin Problems

(See Chapter 4 for more details.)

- **Contact dermatitis** is a rash, which can mimic eczema, caused when the skin comes into contact with certain irritants and allergens.

- **Hives (urticaria)** are a type of rash known as welts, which can last a few days or months. They can appear anywhere on the body and vary in color and shape.

- **Angioedema** is swelling of the deeper layers of the skin, and can sometimes occur with hives.

All the causes of contact dermatitis are not amenable to testing. Urticaria (hives), like eczema, can be aggravated by nonallergic factors, such as heat and viral infections.

FOOD ALLERGIES

Symptoms

One of the first signs of a food allergy is often hives around the mouth, although they may be noticeable after an additional few minutes throughout the whole body. Subsequent reactions may also include swelling of the lips, eyelids, tongue, and rarely, the scrotum in boys, as well as labored breathing, such as wheezing (lower airway obstruction), hoarseness and inspiratory stridor (upper airway obstruction). In more severe food allergic reactions, a child may experience shock or complete collapse (anaphylactic reactions). Not all of these reactions may be present and the order of appearance may be different.

Symptoms to a food allergy usually occur within a few minutes, but may start as late as two hours after ingesting the allergen. A reaction rarely lasts more than a few hours.

Anaphylactic reactions tend to be more severe in allergic individuals, in asthmatics, and children who occasionally take beta-blockers. The medication (adrenaline) used to treat an anaphylactic reaction may not work as well when children are using beta-blockers.

Triggers

These foods will vary in different countries and cultures, depending on when they're introduced to infants' diets. In North America, the most common foods to cause allergic reactions in children are peanut, milk, egg, as well as soy, wheat, fish and sesame seed. In adults and older children, tree nuts and shellfish are more common, which are usually eaten later in childhood. In other cultures, especially those who live by the ocean, shellfish is eaten at a younger age.

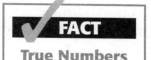

✔ FACT

True Numbers

Twenty-five percent of North Americans claim to have a food allergy, but in reality, only one-third of those are found to have a true food allergy. This works out to 8 percent in infants, 3 to 4 percent in children and 1 to 2 percent in adults.

Diagnosis

There are a series of tests available, from the skin prick test to the ImmunoCap blood test to food challenge tests. (See "What Is Allergy Testing?" on page 32.)

Food-Related Allergies

Food-pollen allergy syndrome

This is also known as oral allergy syndrome (OAS) and fresh-fruit syndrome.

Within a few minutes of eating a fresh fruit, nut, or a raw vegetable, an allergic individual will experience itchiness of the mouth, throat, roof of mouth, and occasionally, vague abdominal discomfort. These symptoms last about 20 to 30 minutes and then disappear spontaneously.

This condition occurs in about 25 to 50 percent of patients with seasonal allergic rhinitis, but may also occur on its own. It's caused by similar allergens that are found in both pollen and some fresh foods. If the fruit has been processed (heated or frozen), symptoms usually don't occur.

Allergy skin tests may confirm the allergy to a fresh fruit or raw vegetable. Your child's allergist will prick the offending fresh food and then your child's skin to get an accurate reading because the protein causing the allergy is only found in the fresh state.

Problem Foods

♦ ♦ ♦ ♦ ♦

Among the foods that commonly cause food-pollen allergy syndrome are:

- Apple
- Peach
- Apricot
- Cherry
- Hazelnut
- Almond
- Melon
- Kiwi
- Banana
- Carrot
- Celery
- Parsnip

Latex-fruit syndrome

Some patients with a latex allergy also have allergies to certain fruits, such as kiwi, water chestnut, avocado, mango, and even to vegetables, such as potato. The main reason: latex and these foods share similar proteins.

People with a latex allergy should be questioned about a fresh-food allergy and vice-versa. If there seems to be a connection, then your child should be tested by an allergist to confirm an allergy.

Food-associated exercise-induced anaphylaxis

Some children will develop anaphylactic reactions after a few minutes of exercise. In 50 percent of cases, such a severe reaction can occur if a child has eaten some food or, more rarely, any meal up to four hours before the physical activity. The same reaction wouldn't occur if either a food wasn't eaten or exercise didn't follow eating.

An allergy skin test may confirm the responsible food, which most commonly may be celery, wheat and shrimp.

ANAPHYLAXIS

Symptoms
At least two body systems must be involved to diagnose an anaphylactic reaction: skin symptoms include hives and swelling; respiratory symptoms include hoarseness, difficulty breathing and wheezing; cardiovascular symptoms include fast heart rate, drop in blood pressure, irregular heartbeat and collapse; and neurological symptoms

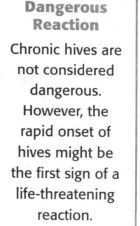

✔ FACT

Dangerous Reaction

Chronic hives are not considered dangerous. However, the rapid onset of hives might be the first sign of a life-threatening reaction.

include coma and, rarely, convulsions. Girls who are post-puberty have increased uterine contractions during an anaphylactic reaction, although they rarely occur.

Triggers
Some causes of this life-threatening reaction are certain foods, especially peanuts, drugs, latex, insect stings, exercise and allergy shots.

Diagnosis
In addition to taking a detailed history of the reaction, your child's allergist will also need to conduct some tests, including urine, blood and skin.

INSECT ALLERGIES

Symptoms
Swelling might occur over the site where the sting occurred. The swelling is not itchy and may last four to seven days. It may also become exaggerated, sometimes extending from the fingers to shoulders, but as long as the swelling is localized, it's not considered dangerous.

An anaphylactic reaction, however, is dangerous. The symptoms, which include hives, difficulty breathing, fast heart rate and, possibly, collapse, occur usually a few minutes (but may be up to two hours) after the sting. (See *Chapter 7: Insect Allergies* for more information.)

Triggers
In North America, the stings of the yellow jacket, wasp, yellow hornet, white-faced hornet and the honeybee account for most of the allergic reactions caused by insects. Rarely, the bite of a deer fly can result in an allergic reaction. In the southern United States, fire ant bites can lead to an allergic reaction.

Ouch!

◆ ◆ ◆ ◆ ◆

Less than
1 percent of
individuals stung
by wasps or bees
have a severe
allergic reaction.

Diagnosis

There are reliable allergy skin tests to determine if an insect allergy exists. They also help to determine the specific venom injections needed to build up a tolerance to the insect venom.

DRUG ALLERGIES

Symptoms/Triggers

Drug allergies usually show up as a rash while a child is taking medication or up to two weeks after stopping a medication. The rash may be hives or a variety of other rashes.

Diagnosis

Allergy skin tests can only accurately confirm a drug allergy to the penicillins.

LATEX ALLERGY

Symptoms

In children, lips can swell or an itchy rash can develop after blowing balloons, or during surgery or a dental procedure. Symptoms may include hives, swelling of the face and difficulty breathing.

Triggers

This allergy tends to occur in individuals who have had numerous surgical procedures, particularly, children with spina bifida or congenital abnormalities of the genito-urinary system. In adults, there tends to be a high incidence among those with certain occupations, such as health-care workers and latex-rubber producers, mainly because of the constant exposure to latex. Children of these workers are also at risk if latex on their work clothing is worn at home and makes contact with the child.

Diagnosis

Allergy tests may confirm a latex allergy.

✔ **FACT**

Nonallergic Reactions

A child can react adversely to a drug for a number of reasons, not just because she's allergic to it. True drug allergies to the penicillins can be confirmed with skin tests.

What Is Allergy Testing?

Testing for allergies is commonly misunderstood. As parents, we'd like to think there's a quick fix to a child's source of discomfort. However, an allergy investigation can't always pinpoint exactly what's causing your child's problem, remove it and cure it. Researchers and allergists have yet to find out why people develop allergic diseases and, therefore, can't prevent nor cure them. We can, however, determine what allergies and irritants exist and help to modify what's happening to a child. Here are some of the methods being used by allergists today.

WHO CAN BE TESTED?

Before any investigation begins, a child's age plays an important role. Children under one year of age can be tested for allergies if they've had a reaction to a specific allergen, such as milk or egg. But, testing for other allergies, such as tree, grass or weed pollens, molds, dust and animals can't be done until a year or two later — it takes until about age two or three before a child's body can develop allergies to such environmental allergens.

For children who have had a life-threatening or anaphylactic reaction, skin testing may also be performed without the risk of a severe reaction — an allergist will normally use watered-down testing materials or dilutions. In such cases, testing becomes very important so that allergic children and parents can take precautions to avoid specific allergens, such as certain foods or insects, and the child can receive a specific allergy shot for the insect allergy.

Born To Be... Allergic?

◆ ◆ ◆ ◆ ◆

Children should not be tested for penicillin or insect allergies just because their parents have these allergies. These allergies are not inherited.

HISTORY-TAKING

One of the first things your doctor will ask is whether you've noted certain situations or circumstances when your child has had a reaction. This will help him identify what is aggravating or triggering the problem. You'll be encouraged to keep a diary when your child has symptoms. Note: reactions commonly occur within minutes after contact with an allergen, or two to four hours after contact with the allergen. Occasionally, they may occur longer after contact; however, a reaction that takes place the next day after contact is usually not related to an allergen.

Here's what to note when your child has a reaction:

✓ Where was your child? At school, outdoors, friend's house, vacation?

✓ What did they contact? Tobacco smoke, perfumes, animals?

✓ What was the weather like? Cold, hot, damp, rapidly changing?

✓ Was your child exercising?

✓ Did he have a cold or flu?

✓ When did these problems first start?

✓ How often do they occur?

✓ How long do they last?

✓ Which seasons of the year are particularly problematic?

✓ What treatments have you tried and which ones were helpful?

✓ Any family members with allergy problems?

Marching In

◆ ◆ ◆ ◆ ◆

Different allergies usually develop at different ages in children. Referred to as the **allergy march**, food allergies and eczema appear in the first 2 years of life. Environmental allergies, such as animal dander, dust, molds and pollens (trees, grasses, weeds), start to appear in children at ages 2 or 3.

ALLERGY SKIN TESTS

Such tests are most widely used by allergists — they're easy, safe, fast and painless. The **skin prick test** is the most common one and it's done by placing drops of a possible allergen extract — trees, grasses, weeds, molds, dust, animals, latex and foods — on the back or forearm. The skin is then lightly pricked with a special needle to absorb the solution, and examined after 15 to 20 minutes to see if there's any redness or swelling. The physician will measure the area — anything larger than 3 mm is considered positive. Testing should be done every few years if the child is experiencing changes.

The **intradermal test** is used when the prick test doesn't provide an answer. The allergen is injected into the outer skin layer with a very fine needle — a swelling will form and is measured. These tests are overly sensitive and could identify allergens that may not be affecting your child, therefore, require careful interpretation by your doctor. They're routinely used in drug and insect testing, but not for testing food allergies.

BLOOD TESTS

The **radioallergosorbent test** (**RAST**) measures the level of a specific antibody called IgE, which the body produces in response to specific antigens like ragweed or grass pollen. It's used when skin testing is not an option, such as when the child has severe eczema or can't stop taking medications, such as antihistamines, that would interfere with skin testing. A blood sample is taken and mixed with the suspecting allergen in a lab to determine any reaction. However, it's not as accurate as a skin test.

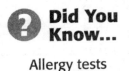

Did You Know...

Allergy tests should be interpreted by a trained professional in the context of the history given by the patient.

The **ImmunoCap** is a newer version of the RAST; however, it still isn't as accurate as a skin test. It's often used together with the skin test to help determine if a patient has lost her sensitivity to a food before taking a food challenge test. More research is being conducted to determine its role in the evaluation of an allergic individual.

Special Measures

Other blood tests are available, but they're seldom used. One of them measures the *eosinophil*, a specialized blood cell that may be elevated in allergic children. Another measures the total amount of IgE antibody in a blood sample. (IgE antibodies may suggest the presence of allergies.) Both tests, however, can't pinpoint which substance may be causing an allergic reaction or its severity. Elevated levels of eosinophil and IgE may also be associated with other disorders not related to allergies.

FOOD CHALLENGE TEST

> ### Don't Self-diagnose
>
> ◆ ◆ ◆ ◆ ◆
>
> In all cases, parents should discuss the best approach for diagnosing a food allergy with the child's allergist.

Food challenges are being used more frequently when the diagnosis is doubtful or there's a chance that a child may be losing the allergy. In a medical facility where treatment can be administered if necessary, the child is fed increasing amounts of the suspect food. If the child can tolerate an amount equal to a full serving, then the food can be added back into the diet.

Other types of challenges are also used mainly for research purposes. They include injecting the allergen in question directly into the nose or lung and measuring the breathing responses with special devices.

Elimination diets, which involve eliminating a suspect food, can be done for one to two weeks. If there's an improvement, the food can be added back

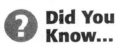
into a child's diet. If multiple foods are involved, a more severe elimination diet may be prescribed and foods added back one at a time. Such diets, which are not frequently recommended, can be dangerous because they can cause nutritional problems.

Other approaches may include keeping a food journal, however, it may be confusing especially if other nonfood causes are involved.

ASTHMA TESTS

Pulmonary function tests frequently show normal results in symptom-free patients. In order to determine whether a patient is asthmatic, he's asked to inhale a broncho-constricting agent, such as methacholine. If a patient is wheezing at the time of the test, there may be an obstruction to breathing, particularly on expiration (breathing out).

A **chest X-ray** is performed primarily to rule out other diseases that can mimic asthma, such as a foreign body, a birth abnormality of a major blood vessel, cystic fibrosis or a chest mass. Occasionally, asthma can be detected in chest X-rays.

Your child's physician might conduct a **sweat test** to rule out cystic fibrosis. The test measures salts in your child's sweat. While cystic fibrosis affects many of the body's symptoms, it can mimic similar symptoms caused by asthma and allergies.

CONTROVERSIAL TESTING

You may have heard of other 'new-age' tests available to test the presence of an allergy in your child. To date, the ones you'll learn about in this section haven't been proven scientifically and are largely experimental. Some of them may have been performed by independent researchers in controlled clinical trials but have been untested by credible scientific studies. Other tests have been helpful in understanding other diseases aside from allergic conditions. Here are the four most popular alternative tests:

1. Cytotoxic Test

White blood cells (cells used by the body to fight infection) are separated from the rest of the blood and then mixed with sterile water and serum. This mixture is then placed on a microscope slide coated with a dried preparation of the allergen. The cells are then examined at intervals that can last up to two hours for any structural changes in cells. However, there is no scientific evidence that a food allergy causes any changes in white blood cell shape, nor is there any proof that changes in the structure of white cells has anything to do with food allergy. The changes that occur in this procedure could easily be blamed on other factors, such as temperature of the solution, length of time in the solution, or certain contaminants.

2. Provocation-Neutralization

The aim of this procedure is to expose the patient to doses of various allergens intradermally (into the skin), subcutaneously (under the skin), or sublingually (under the tongue), in order to produce any kind of change. Increasing doses of allergens are

---

Testing Fears

◆ ◆ ◆ ◆ ◆

An allergy test can help determine what's likely causing your child's debilitating symptoms. Allergy testing is safe — for example, in skin tests only a small, diluted sample of a possible allergen is used to ensure there isn't a severe reaction.

Prevention Testing

◆ ◆ ◆ ◆ ◆

For many years, researchers have conducted tests to determine if allergies can be prevented. For the latest findings, see *Chapter 12: Prevention of Allergies.*

administered to the patient by one of the three different routes mentioned on the previous page, at 10-minute intervals, until a symptom occurs. Once a symptom is present, that dose is known as the provocative or positive dose. The dose is then gradually lowered at 10-minute intervals until there are no symptoms — that dose is known as the neutralizing dose, which is used for treating the diverse symptoms experienced when eating the food. There are no standardized protocols or particular set of symptoms researchers use as guidelines. Instead, any subjective sensation, such as lightheadedness, irritability, excessive gas, or any unusual feeling could be considered a symptom of the allergens. There also is no scientific basis or results for this procedure.

3. Electrodermal Testing (Vega Test)

This method uses a galvanometer that measures electrical activity of the skin at specific acupuncture points. The patient holds the negative electrode, while a probe held at a specific skin acupuncture point maintains the positive electrode. Points on the lower extremities of the body are more specific for food allergy; points on the upper extremities and trunk are more specific to inhalant allergy; and points on the scalp tend to be associated with rhinitis and sinusitis. The patient is diagnosed as having an allergy if the probe shows a drop in electrical current when it touches a specific point. The device spews out a computerized readout of the 'allergies' it finds. This procedure is currently very popular in Europe. Again, there is no scientific support for the validity of this procedure.

4. Applied Kinesiology

This test measures a patient's muscle strength to determine a possible allergy. The patient holds in one hand a container filled with a specific allergen while a technician measures the muscle strength in the other arm. Weaker muscle strength while holding the allergen indicates an allergy to the substance being held. When uncooperative infants are being tested, the mother will hold the infant's hand while the muscle strength of her other hand is measured before and while holding her child's hand. The results are usually not reproducible and often bizarre.

Magic Potions?

Given the limitations of skin and blood testing, it's understandable for concerned parents to search for answers to a child's allergy. However, at present, there are no magic tests that can accurately pinpoint a person's allergy problem.

Proceed With Caution

You should be wary of allergy tests that…

• …give long lists of foods that might be causing your child's allergy or that ask you to score the severity of the reaction. Individuals with true food allergies are usually only allergic to a few foods, usually less than five.

• …attempt to determine the severity of an allergic problem. Food reactions depend on many factors, such as the state of the food (fresh or cooked), the amount eaten, the health of the individual, etc. Even if a reaction is mild initially there's no guarantee that a future exposure won't cause a more serious reaction.

PART 2

Allergic Conditions

Chapter 2

ASTHMA

Breathing Disorder of the Lungs

ASTHMA HAS BEEN A RECOGNIZED ILLNESS since the time of the ancient Greeks. The term 'asthma' is derived from the Greek word *aenai*, meaning "short-drawn breath" or "panting." Despite medical advances and improved therapies, there has been an increase in the frequency of the disease. It's not clear why, but early diagnosis and aggressive treatment can improve its outcome.

Does My Child Have Asthma?

◆ ◆ ◆ ◆ ◆

If you suspect your child has asthma, watch for the following symptoms. They'll either recur many times during the year or persist for weeks or months:

• Coughing

• Shortness of breath

• Wheezing

WHAT IS ASTHMA?

Asthma is a disease that causes the muscles around the bronchial tubes (airways) in the lungs to contract, as well as the lining of the bronchial tubes to become inflamed and swollen. This inflammation involves many different white cells, which release very potent chemicals and invade the tube lining. It produces a thick mucus, causing the airways to become narrow, very 'twitchy' and sensitive, and consequently respond easily to triggers such as colds, exercise and strong odors.

Asthma Symptoms

We often associate asthma with a number of symptoms, in particular, wheezing. However, the common misconception that a person must wheeze in order to have asthma is unfounded. In fact, many patients with asthma not only wheeze, but instead have other symptoms. These are:

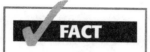

FACT

ER Visits

Asthma is the No. 1 cause of hospital emergency visits and school absenteeism.

Ageless Asthma

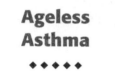

Your child can develop asthma at any age, at any time, although it's more common in childhood.

Persistent cough. Typically, these patients will catch a cold and develop chest congestion with a night and early morning cough, as well as cough with exertion. The cough worsens when a sufferer is exposed to cold air, is laughing or talking on the phone, among other factors, and it can linger for weeks or months. The cough *does not* respond to cough medicine or antibiotics.

Shortness of breath. Asthma patients complain of shortness of breath with minimal activity, such as climbing stairs or walking outside in cold weather. Frequently, both patients and doctors unknowingly attribute this symptom to lack of physical fitness rather than to asthma.

Wheezing. Spasm of the bronchial tubes causes a tightening or narrowing of the airways. This creates a particular whistling sound that may be heard by the patient or the doctor when he listens through a stethoscope. Wheezing can be associated with a feeling of chest tightness, gasping and difficulty breathing.

Asthma Numbers

According to the most current Health Canada research, 12.2 percent of children were diagnosed with asthma. The incidence of asthma is probably higher due to underdiagnosis. In the U.S., the American Academy of Allergy, Asthma & Immunology estimates that asthma affects about five million children.

Asthma in Stages

1. ASTHMA IN INFANCY

In the past, asthma was not diagnosed in babies. Typically, these infants will have a 'rattly chest,' especially following a viral infection like a cold, and it will persist for a long time after a cold. They may also experience persistent coughing, wheezing or shortness of breath, and there's either a family history of asthma, allergies and eczema or they also have eczema and/or food allergies.

2. ASTHMA IN CHILDHOOD

During early childhood, the most common trigger for asthma is a viral infection like a cold, which tends to trigger persistent coughing. Young children don't often complain about shortness of breath, but during physical activity they tend to be slower than their peers — some children avoid exercise altogether. Decreased physical activity can contribute to these children becoming overweight. In late childhood, colds and other factors, such as allergies, can trigger asthma.

The Allergy Connection

◆ ◆ ◆ ◆ ◆

Asthma is associated with environmental allergies in most children over the age of 6 who have the disease.

Don't Ignore Inflammation

Treating inflammation, even in very mild asthma, is crucial. If inflammation goes untreated, it can cause chronic changes, such as scarring of the lungs. Special medication known as anti-inflammatories help reduce or control inflammation. (See "Asthma Medications" on page 52 for more details.)

3. ASTHMA IN ADOLESCENTS AND ADULTS

In addition to a persistent cough, shortness of breath and wheezing, adolescents and adults may complain of chest pain, which often results in a referral to a heart specialist to rule out cardiovascular problems. Once it's determined there is no heart condition, a doctor is typically successful treating the chest pain with asthma medications. Although asthma symptoms can be present for many years, the condition can go undiagnosed until adulthood.

Common Triggers

We know what can cause an asthma attack, but it's still unclear why certain people will develop the inflammation that causes asthma. Both allergies and certain irritants can trigger asthma in your child, either on their own or in combination. A physician will evaluate patients for certain allergies and recommend caregivers create an environment that avoids common allergens and irritants.

Allergens	Irritants	Other Triggers
• Animal dander	• Cigarette smoke; smoke from a fireplace or wood stove	• Extreme weather (cold, hot, dry, humid)
• Dust and dust mites		• Viral infections (colds or the flu)
• Molds	• Smog	
• Pollen (trees, grass, weeds)	• Chemicals, strong odors, sprays	• Exercise
		• Medications with aspirin. Acetaminophen (Tylenol, Tempra) is a better choice

Asthma Or Something Else?

Certain conditions in children can mimic asthma — including pneumonia, inhaled foreign bodies, cystic fibrosis, structural abnormalities at birth and an immune deficiency. In adults, lung infections, chronic lung disease from smoking, heart problems, acid reflux and chest tumors may mask themselves as asthma. Your child's doctor will confirm asthma by taking a detailed history and specialized tests.

Making A Diagnosis

TOP 5 METHODS

❓ Did You Know...

It can take up to 8 weeks for the swelling and inflammation in your child's airways to decrease after an asthma attack.

1. One of the most important steps in making an asthma diagnosis in your child is taking a *detailed medical history* to assess a patient's symptoms, associated allergies and possible irritants in the home.

2. Detailed physical examination by the child's physician to assess whether there is any wheezing or rapid breathing.

3. Allergy testing and evaluation, if indicated by the history.

4. Additional testing: a chest X-ray can help to rule out other diseases that mimic asthma.

5. Breathing tests, such as a pulmonary function test, can be conducted before and after a child takes a bronchodilator (medication that helps expand the bronchial airway) to help confirm the diagnosis. Further breathing tests known as a metacholine or histamine challenge can be done if the diagnosis is still uncertain. However, both tests can be negative even when asthma is

present. Therefore, if asthma is strongly suspected and tests are inconclusive, your child's physician may recommend a trial of asthma treatment.

How Bad Is It?

To help the doctor determine the severity of your child's asthma, know the answers to these questions on your next visit:

- How many days has she missed in school?
- What symptoms does she experience during the day and at night?
- What kind of physical activity does she do?
- How many times has she been rushed to the hospital?
- What/how much medication is she using?

Managing Asthma

The objective in treating asthma successfully is to control the inflammation process so your child can lead a completely normal life. Here are the main goals:

- No symptoms
- Normal activities with no restrictions
- Minimal or no flare-ups
- No hospital or emergency room visits
- No absence from school or work due to asthma
- Minimal or no medications
- No side effects from medications

Exercise and Asthma

◆ ◆ ◆ ◆ ◆

There are many benefits to regular exercise — among them, making your lungs more efficient. Talk to your child's doctor about developing an exercise regimen.

BREATHING EASIER — HOW TO:

One of the most important factors in managing asthma is reducing inflammation when possible. To do this, parents should limit exposure to allergens, as well as irritants. Many studies have shown that reducing or eliminating certain allergens significantly reduces asthma symptoms and the need for less medication to control the disease. Here are a few tips on how to minimize exposure. (For more tips on reducing allergens, see *Chapter 11: Environmental Control*.)

Dust and dust mite control

✓ Remove all dust collectors, such as stuffed toys, from the bedroom.

✓ Keep humidity at 30 to 50 percent and temperature at 20 degrees Celsius/68 degrees Fahrenheit.

✓ Remove carpets, especially in bedroom and play areas.

✓ Encase mattresses, box springs and pillows with zippered allergy-proof covers.

✓ Choose washable bedding and launder it once a week in hot water to kill dust mites.

✓ Vacuum/clean floors, mattresses and window coverings regularly. Don't vacuum when your allergic child is in the room. Instead, wait about half an hour for the dust to settle.

Animal control

✓ Remove furry pets from the home, if possible. Otherwise, keep pets out of your child's bedroom and the car.

✓ Wash pets every week.

Double Dose

♦ ♦ ♦ ♦ ♦

The two main components of treating asthma include:

1. Controlling allergens and irritants

2. Taking asthma medications

✓ Don't replace a pet when it dies, or choose pets that don't shed hair, such as reptiles or turtles.

Pollen control

✓ Keep windows/doors closed during high pollen counts.

✓ Use an air conditioner during summer months.

✓ Keep garden clothing out of the house.

Mold control

Molds are fungi that produce spores that can be inhaled. Both indoor and outdoor molds can aggravate asthma in sensitive individuals.

✓ Keep humidity in the home between 30 and 50 percent and indoor temperature at 20 degrees Celsius/68 degrees Fahrenheit.

✓ Remove items that can increase molds in the home, such as, plants, aquariums, etc.

✓ Clean ventilation equipment and replace filters regularly.

✓ Use exhaust fans in bathrooms and when cooking to reduce the growth of mold.

✓ Wash windows and shower stalls with bleach.

Irritant control

✓ Avoid smoking in the home.

✓ Avoid using a fireplace and wood stoves.

✓ Avoid paint fumes, house renovations and strong odors from household cleaners, air fresheners and perfumes/deodorants, especially when the asthma is not controlled.

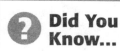

Did You Know...

Stress has been attributed to making asthma symptoms worse, especially if your child's asthma isn't well controlled.

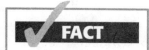

FACT

Soothing the Side Effects

Inhaled corticosteroids, which are used to control inflammation, have few side effects that can be effectively minimized.

ASTHMA MEDICATIONS

There are two main groups of asthma medications: **bronchodilators** and **anti-inflammatories**. Both can be either inhaled or taken orally.

Bronchodilators

This class of medication helps to open the bronchial tubes by relaxing the muscles that surround them. They only help to reduce the acute symptoms of asthma, such as wheezing, coughing and shortness of breath, but they do not help to control the inflammation — that's what anti-inflammatories are for. Several groups of bronchodilators are available:

Short-acting beta agonists (Ventolin, Bricanyl, Alupent, etc.) — work within minutes and their effects last between four to six hours.

Long-acting beta agonists (Oxeze, Serevent) — last for up to 12 hours. Currently, both medications are not recommended for controlling acute symptoms, but rather as a combination therapy with inhaled corticosteroids (anti-inflammatories).

Theophylline drugs (Choledyl, Theo-Dur, Somephilline 12) — oral medications frequently used in the past. Because of numerous serious side effects, and the availability of better medications, these drugs are rarely used today.

Atropine-like medications (Atrovent) — relieves the spasm of the bronchial tubes and is used primarily in the emergency room when short-acting beta agonists aren't sufficient to control an acute attack.

Asthma Checkup

◆ ◆ ◆ ◆ ◆

Here's a quick tip to determine whether your child's asthma is under control: he has no need, or very little need (2 to 3 times a week) for a 'quick fix' from the bronchodilator.

Anti-inflammatories

This class of medication is the mainstay of asthma treatment. In order to successfully treat asthma, your child's doctor will attempt to control or eliminate the inflammation so that airways are less 'twitchy' and asthma symptoms under control. By controlling inflammation, you'll minimize your child's need for bronchodilators.

Anti-inflammatory medications are divided into two groups: **corticosteroid** or **non-corticosteroid** medications.

Corticosteroid Medications

1. **Oral corticosteroids** (Prednisone, Pediapred) — are one of the most effective anti-inflammatories available. However, because of numerous serious side effects when used for long periods (more than 14 days), they're not an option for maintenance therapy. A short course of oral corticosteroids (five to 10 days) can be very effective in providing dramatic relief of acute asthma symptoms with minimal or no side effects.

2. **Inhaled corticosteroids** (Flovent, Pulmicort, QVAR) — are very effective anti-inflammatory agents, with minimal side effects when used at the recommended dose. Common side effects are reversible and include hoarseness and thrush (fungal infection), which can be minimized by rinsing the mouth and throat with water immediately after taking the medication and also using a spacer device, such as an aerochamber.

    The dosage can be adjusted according to the patient's condition. When using inhaled corticosteroids, ensure your child's doctor regularly follows her progress.

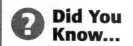 **Did You Know...**

When medication is inhaled through a puffer it travels directly to the lungs more quickly, where it's needed.

Non-corticosteroid Medications

1. **Intal and Tilade** — are effective anti-inflammatory medications that were regularly used years ago. While these inhaled medications are not corticosteroids, they are weaker than inhaled corticosteroids and must be taken frequently (up to four times a day), which reduces the effectiveness because a patient is less likely to comply.

2. **Zaditen** — an oral medication approved in Canada for treating asthma. (It is not approved in the United States.) However, its effectiveness in controlling asthma is debatable. Its anti-inflammatory and anti-histamine effect may also be beneficial in certain skin problems.

3. **Leukotrienes antagonist** (Singulair, Accolate) — a group of medications given orally as tablets. They specifically target the inflammation and can be either used on their own in mild asthma cases, or as an add-on therapy to inhaled corticosteroids in moderate or severe asthma cases. They are very safe, as well as effective, in a select group of patients. They can be used in adults and children as young as two years old.

4. **Combination therapies** (Advair, Symbicort) — medications that combine an inhaled corticosteroid and a long-acting bronchodilator in one device (Diskus, Turbuhaler). They can be effective when the use of an inhaled corticosteroid is not sufficient to control a child's asthma. However, they should *not* be used as a first-line medication therapy.

✔ **FACT**

Breathing In Benefits

One advantage to taking an inhaled corticosteroid over an oral medication is that it doesn't filter through other body systems, so it generally causes less side effects.

Asthma Action Plan

Develop an action plan with your child's doctor to help him control his asthma. The written plan guides you and your child on what to do to manage asthma every day, and when to increase medications to regulate flare-ups. Some patients will find it useful to keep a daily diary or to use a peak flow meter, which is a device for self-monitoring the status of the asthma.

ASTHMA FACTS — Q & A

Q: Can my child outgrow asthma?

A: Yes, about 25 percent of children no longer experience asthma symptoms as they get older. However, symptoms in some children can return as they get older.

Q: Is there a cure for my child's asthma?

A: No, there is no cure for the condition. However, asthma can be controlled by avoiding allergens and triggers and taking medication and your child can lead a normal, active life.

Q: Will exercise make my child's asthma worse?

A: There are a few things your child can do to avoid making his asthma worse during exercise: do warm-up exercises at the start of any physical activity and cool-down exercises at the end. Your child's doctor may recommend she take asthma medicine 15 to 20 minutes before exercising.

Q: Are inhaled steroids safe?

A: The steroids that are used to treat asthma are called corticosteroids. They're generally considered safe and very effective in controlling your child's asthma. These steroids are not to be confused with anabolic steroids used by some athletes. Use them as directed by your child's physician to ensure best results.

RHINITIS

Upper Airway Disorders

YOUR CHILD IS CONSTANTLY FIGHTING THE sniffles and sneezes, the watery, itchy eyes and a sore throat. Seems like a string of occurrences of the common cold. But before you reach for relief from the medicine cabinet, you need to make sure you know what you're fighting. Symptoms of a cold often mimic other conditions grouped up under a large category we call rhinitis.

Rhinitis refers to a reddened and swollen lining of the nose, or inflammation of the mucous membrane of the nose. There are several forms of rhinitis caused by a number of different factors, one of which is the virus also responsible for the common cold, but allergy-causing substances called allergens cause other forms of rhinitis. Here, in this chapter, you will learn about a number of different types of rhinitis, both allergic and nonallergic.

Rhinitis Resolve

◆ ◆ ◆ ◆ ◆

The good news is that in both seasonal allergic rhinitis and perennial allergic rhinitis, simple allergy skin tests can detect the suspected allergens.

WHAT IS ALLERGIC RHINITIS?

If your child is experiencing symptoms only at certain times of the year, like spring, summer or fall, he probably has **seasonal allergic rhinitis**. Pollens (trees, grasses, or weeds) or outdoor molds are the prime culprits. But if your child is suffering year-round symptoms, indoor allergens, such as house dust mites, indoor molds and animal dander may be responsible for his condition, which experts call **perennial allergic rhinitis** or **year-round indoor allergies**.

Hay Fever: When The Nose Knows

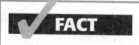

FACT

Achew on This

Approximately 75 percent of seasonal allergic rhinitis is caused by ragweed, 40 percent by grass and 9 percent by trees.

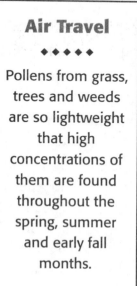

Air Travel

◆ ◆ ◆ ◆ ◆

Pollens from grass, trees and weeds are so lightweight that high concentrations of them are found throughout the spring, summer and early fall months.

Seasonal allergic rhinitis is commonly known as 'hay fever' or 'rose fever.' The two terms were first used in the 19th century because it was believed that symptoms related to hay or flowers, like the rose. Today we recognize that hay is not a major cause and that fever is not a symptom of the condition. Hay fever affects approximately 20 percent of individuals; up to 40 percent of children are affected. Here's what someone suffering from seasonal allergic rhinitis or hay fever will experience:

A runny nose. Watery clear liquid, produced by the swelling in the nasal membrane, can run intermittently or continually from a child's nose. Even though helping your child clear his nose can be helpful, this will only offer temporary relief. The swelling will continue to produce secretions. Sometimes, the mucus may run into the back of the throat causing irritation, dryness and coughing.

Itching. The inside of a child's nose may become irritated, resulting in a 'rabbit nose' reaction — frequent twitching of the nose to relieve irritation. She may also push the tip of her nose upwards to help open the nose to allow for better breathing — a movement called the 'allergic salute.' A child might also develop a line on the bridge of the nose from these frequent movements known as the 'allergic crease.'

Sneezing. You'll hear it frequently, especially in the morning. It can be quite draining for many young sufferers. It's produced when the chemicals released during an allergic reaction irritate the nerve endings in the nose lining.

Histamine Comes From...

◆ ◆ ◆ ◆ ◆

Histamine is found in a particular type of cell known as mast cells, which are found in the lining of the nose, lungs, skin and intestines. When an allergen makes contact with a mast cell, it releases histamine and causes an allergic reaction.

Congestion (stuffiness). This develops due to swelling of the nose lining. A frequently congested nose will lead to mouth breathing, which can also cause a dry throat since the mouth isn't able to humidify the air like the nose. To clear the congestion, sufferers may clear their throats or begin coughing. At nighttime, you may hear snoring, which could disturb a child's sleep and lead to fatigue and irritability during the day. This congestion can affect both nose openings or only one side and can alternate from one side to the other.

Other symptoms:

Decreased sense of smell and taste. This happens because of a combination of factors that affect the nose and throat.

Nose bleeds caused by ruptured blood vessels near the irritated lining.

Changes in the bones of the face such as an overgrowth of the upper jaw (overbite) and elongation of the face (allergic facies) due to prolonged obstruction.

Dark color patches (allergic shiners) around the eyes and nose. The color changes are caused by obstructed blood flow around the nose and, in particular, under the eyes from the congestion and not because of lack of sleep or rest.

Beyond The Nose

Other areas may also be affected by allergic rhinitis.

Sinus cavities. The nose leads into these cavities, which are actually holes in the skull. These can become filled with mucus, resulting in sinus headaches or infections.

Adenoids. Similar to the tonsils, they're located at the back of the nose and can also become irritated and swollen. If the swelling causes a significant obstruction to breathing, the adenoids may need to be removed surgically.

Eyes. May become swollen, red, teary and itchy.

Ears. May become itchy, scratchy and irritated. They may feel blocked with fluid or infection; hearing may be muffled.

Throat. May become sore and can result in clearing or coughing.

Undercover Mold

◆ ◆ ◆ ◆ ◆

Mold spores can harbor in:

• Piles of plant clippings left in moist, warm weather

• Rotting wood

• Moldy leaves

• Places that are dark and damp and have little airflow

WHAT'S TO BLAME?

Seasonal allergic rhinitis is caused by outdoor mold and pollen, which is produced by grass, trees and weeds in sufficient quantities to affect sensitive individuals. Grass, tree and weed pollens are light and easily carried by the wind. In northern and eastern parts of North America, tree pollen is found in high concentrations from April to June and grass pollen from mid-May to the end of July. Ragweed pollen travels through the air from the second week of August to the first frost in mid- or late October in the same area (although this pattern will vary depending on the geographic location).

Airborne pollen triggers the cells in the lining of the nose to release various chemical mediators, such as histamine. This results in inflammation of the nose lining, which causes increased mucus production and swelling to produce the reactions listed on the previous pages.

Outdoor airborne mold spores, such as alternaria and cladosporium, are also a common cause of allergic rhinitis and have been implicated as a significant trigger of allergic asthma (see *Chapter 2: Asthma* for more information).

LIMIT EXPOSURE

Avoiding triggers is the best medicine for hay fever, but keeping a child from playing outdoors all the time is impossible. For this reason, parents need to practice a two-pronged approach:

1. Controlling the indoor air environment

2. Reducing exposure to pollens outdoors

(See *Chapter 11: Environmental Control* for specific steps on controlling the indoor air environment and reducing your child's exposure to allergens.)

Pollen Producers

◆ ◆ ◆ ◆ ◆

The following are the most common allergy-producing pollen in the north-eastern part of the U.S. and Canada:

• Trees: birch, elm, maple

• Timothy grass

• Short and giant ragweed

These types of pollen will vary depending on the geographical location.

Flower Power

Unlike ragweed, flowers and goldenrod don't normally cause allergies. Their pollens are heavy and sticky, which means they're not likely to become airborne like lighter-weight weed or tree pollens. Flower and goldenrod pollen rely on insects, such as bees and butterflies, to carry their pollens.

? **Did You Know...**

There are many forms of rhinitis. While nonallergic rhinitis has similar symptoms to the allergic form, it can be caused by a host of different factors, including infections, structural problems in the nose, and even some medications.

Perennial Allergic Rhinitis

Unlike seasonal allergic rhinitis, which generally disappears after the first frost, sufferers of perennial allergic rhinitis will still complain of congestion and a runny nose year-round. That's because this form of rhinitis is caused by indoor allergens, such as house dust mites, animal dander and indoor molds and cockroaches, which may be detected by allergy skin tests. Sufferers of perennial allergic rhinitis experience similar symptoms to those of seasonal allergic rhinitis. (See "Allergy-proofing Your Home" on page 67 for ways to minimize indoor allergens.) There are also agents in your own home that can aggravate your child's allergies. The most offensive irritants include cleansers and detergents, tobacco smoke, cooking odors, paint fumes, perfumes and dry air.

Indoor Allergens

A child's own environment could be partly to blame for his allergic reactions.

Culprits	Where Are They Found?
House dust mites	in overstuffed furniture, bedding/pillows, carpeting, stuffed toys
Animal dander	from cats, dogs and other pets
Indoor molds	in trash cans, refrigerator drip pan, shower curtains, plants, aquariums, furnace/ventilation equipment and filters, basement (around pipes)
Cockroaches	in inner city homes and schools, mainly in kitchens and bathrooms

Nonallergic Rhinitis

Sensitivities to pollen, mold or dust aren't the only cause of rhinitis. Irritants such as cigarette smoke, perfumes, paint smells, and extremes of cold, hot or damp weather can bring on an irritated nose and throat. Even viral infections, such as the one that causes the common cold and flu, can make your nose miserable for an extended period. Sometimes these same irritants can also aggravate those who have allergic rhinitis problems. Certain medications and various changes in the nose or surrounding parts, like the adenoids, may create similar problems. Allergy skin tests will not detect any of these causes. Here's a breakdown of the main causes:

INFECTIONS

The culprits here are viruses and bacteria. The common cold is an example of a viral infection. Sometimes it's difficult for parents to distinguish a cold or flu from an episode of allergic rhinitis. If your child has a low-grade fever, for example, she most likely has the common cold. With a bacterial infection, patients will complain about feeling stuffy and a thick greenish mucus (discharge) will ooze from the nose.

The infection can also spread into the sinus cavities (sinusitis) and cause headaches. If your child's doctor finds more than one infection or doesn't see any improvement after three to four weeks, he may order X-rays to look for other causes, such as enlarged adenoids or structural changes in the nose or sinuses that would prevent infections

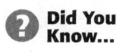

Did You Know...

Children under 2 years old are likely to catch between 5 and 9 colds a year; those between 3 and 5 years typically catch 3 to 4 colds, compared to older children and adults who usually get 1 to 2 a year. That's because children tend to spend more time with other affected children, and their immune systems aren't as developed.

from clearing up. In a rare minority of cases, blood tests may also be required to determine whether a child's defense systems (immune system) have any deficiencies that would allow such infections to take hold so easily.

STRUCTURAL PROBLEMS

There could be several problems in the body that can cause a flare-up of rhinitis. Among them are:

- *Enlarged adenoids,* one of the most common problems among young children.

- *The septum,* a child's middle nose bone, can be twisted or off-center, causing an obstructed air passage in the nose. If the condition is severe, surgery may be necessary; however, it's usually performed when the child is older and the bones are more formed.

- *Polyps or outgrowths* of the nasal lining may also block a child's nasal passage. Although they're more common in adults, in rare instances, their presence in children may indicate cystic fibrosis.

- *Tumors* may exist in very rare situations.

- *Tiny hairs or cilia,* which line the nasal passages, can be involved in an even more rare condition. The cilia regularly filter unwanted particles such as dust or smoke that reach the area. When they aren't doing their job properly, the area can become infected. These patients usually also experience chest infections. The condition is diagnosed by taking a piece of the nose lining (biopsy) and examining it under a microscope.

Foreign Passenger

◆ ◆ ◆ ◆ ◆

Don't discount a foreign object causing an obstruction of airflow — children may push certain objects into the nose, such as gum, crayons or marbles. If this is the case, you'll notice a foul-smelling discharge from the blocked nostril.

VASOMOTOR RHINITIS

This form of rhinitis is neither allergic nor infectious. It develops from an imbalance of the systems that regulate the nose lining, including the nerves and blood vessels within the nose. Sudden changes in temperature, humidity or moisture, as well as strong irritating odors from tobacco smoke, paint smells and perfumes, can cause such problems. They can even further irritate the child who has an allergic nose.

MEDICATIONS

Over-the-counter nose sprays, such as Otrivin, may give you quick relief, but can cause a condition known as *rhinitis medicamentosa* if the medication is overused. Therefore, it's not recommended that such medications be used for more than one week.

Finding Relief

Before you run to the drugstore for a quick fix, see your doctor about a proper diagnosis. He'll take your child's medical history, assess her physical findings and order appropriate tests, such as skin tests or a blood RAST (see *Chapter 1: Introduction to Allergies* for details). Based on those findings, he'll recommend the appropriate treatment. Most importantly in the treatment of rhinitis, primarily with allergic individuals, is avoiding identifiable causes or irritants (see *Chapter 11: Environmental Control* for more information), the use of appropriate medications and allergy shots (immunotherapy).

Vitamin Power?

◆ ◆ ◆ ◆ ◆

There's no evidence vitamins can help fight specific allergies. Instead, allergists recommend they be considered as part of a healthy diet.

ENVIRONMENTAL CONTROLS: ALLERGY-PROOFING YOUR HOME

Minimizing exposure to allergens and irritants is one of your best defenses against a rhinitis reaction. Here are some sure-fire ways to do that: (For a more detailed list, see *Chapter 11, Environmental Control.*)

✓ Clean an allergic child's bedroom at least twice a week.

✓ Encase pillows and mattresses with special allergy-proof covers.

✓ Wash sheets and pillowcases at least once a week in hot water. Wash mattress covers and blankets regularly, too.

✓ Remove all mold and dust collectors, such as stuffed animals and books, from bedroom or other rooms where children spend lots of time. Or, ensure these items are washed regularly and stored away.

✓ Clean and vacuum rugs, upholstered furniture, mattresses and curtains regularly.

✓ Clean furnace filters regularly.

✓ Get your furnace and air-conditioning units serviced once a year. Well-maintained units have been found to reduce pollen and mold counts.

✓ Don't smoke in the home or around children.

✓ Avoid painting in the home while an allergic child is present or, if necessary, ensure the area is well-ventilated.

✓ Avoid cleansers with heavy perfumes or noxious fumes that aggravate symptoms.

Filtering Filters

◆ ◆ ◆ ◆ ◆

The jury is still out on whether specially designed filters, such as a HEPA filter, can minimize dust and pollen in the home or workplace.

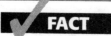 **FACT**

Flooring Fix

Find an alternative flooring to carpets in your home. Carpets can trap allergy-causing substances like dust mites and mold.

✓ Regulate the household humidity at less than 50 percent, which can be measured with a hygrometer, available at most local hardware stores. Too much humidity may cause an overgrowth of mold in the home.

✓ Keep windows closed during the pollen season. Window air conditioners may help filter pollen.

MEDICAL TREATMENT

Allergic and irritant rhinitis can be treated using antihistamines, decongestants and topical nose sprays. Immunotherapy is more specific for allergic rhinitis.

Antihistamines. Refers to a group of drugs that block the effects of histamines, one of the natural chemicals the body releases into the tissues and body fluids during an allergic reaction. For this reason, they're most effective before exposure to an allergen or at the start of the allergy season, but they're also useful once symptoms have started. Because it can take two to three weeks before being effective, antihistamines are best used on a regular basis for a few weeks or months rather then as needed for one or two days only. Although the optimal antihistamines control symptoms and cause few side effects, some may cause drowsiness, dizziness and dry mouth. However, many patients acclimate to antihistamine side effects and these become minimal with continued use. Newer varieties of antihistamines have been developed to cause few or no side effects. They include Claritin (loratadine), Reactine (ceterizine), Allegra (fexofenadine) and Aeirus (desloratadine).

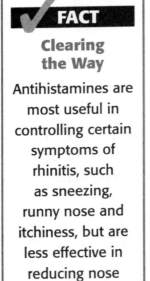

✓ FACT

Clearing the Way

Antihistamines are most useful in controlling certain symptoms of rhinitis, such as sneezing, runny nose and itchiness, but are less effective in reducing nose stuffiness.

Doctor Call

◆ ◆ ◆ ◆ ◆

With a variety of treatment options available to treat rhinitis, call your child's physician first, before choosing any over-the-counter medication.

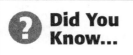

Did You Know...

Don't expect a quick fix for your child's allergic rhinitis with nasal corticosteroid sprays. While they're very effective, they can take up to three weeks to show improvement.

Decongestants. These come in topical and oral forms, shrinking the blood vessels in the nose to reduce congestion and may be used together with antihistamines. Topical drugs, such as Otrivin or Neo-Synephrine, narrows the blood vessels, which in turn cuts down on nasal swelling. However, prolonged use for more than a couple of weeks can lead to a rebound effect, producing excessive swelling called *rhinitis medicamentosa*. For this reason, oral decongestants, such as Sudafed, can also relieve congestion without the same effects. They, however, have other side effects, including irritability, headaches, insomnia and an elevation in blood pressure and rapid heart rates or palpitations. Prolonged use of these drugs is also not recommended.

Nasal corticosteroid sprays. Sprays that contain corticosteroids are the most effective medications in treating allergic rhinitis. These help control inflammation by decreasing the swelling of the nose lining and reducing the nasal discharge — without the rebound effect of topical decongestants. This, in turn, helps to decrease the sensitivity of the nose not only to allergens, such as pollen and dust, but also to other irritants like perfume, paint fumes and tobacco smoke. You may not notice any improvement in your child's condition for a few days and their full effect may take two to three weeks. There may be local irritation to the nose lining and some bleeding, however, lowering the dosage or using saline sprays before using corticosteroid sprays may help reduce the bleeding.

Spray Stunt

Parents will be relieved to know that one of the side effects of taking oral corticosteroids for a long period — stunted growth in children — is not seen with corticosteroid sprays, as long as they aren't overused. It's recommended your physician monitor their use. Corticosteroid nasal sprays include: Beconase (beclomethasone), Rhinalar (flunisolide), Rhinocort (budesonide), Flonase (fluticasone), Nasonex (mometasone) and Nasacort (triamcinolone).

Oral corticosteroids. Prednisone, for example, may be used for the occasional short course (less than one week) when other therapies become ineffective.

Other nose sprays.

Sodium cromoglycate (Intal) has no corticosteroid properties and can prevent an allergen from releasing mediators such as histamine from the mast cell in the lining of the nose. Like antihistamines, these sprays can be taken before the start of the allergy season and are helpful throughout it.

Levocabastine (Livostin) is a topical antihistamine that can block the effect of histamine. It works fairly well during the allergy season.

Atropine (Atrovent) has a beneficial effect on vasomotor rhinitis where the nose discharge may be brought on by cold air, hot food or certain spices.

Lubricants (Salinex and Rhinaris) are lubricants that are useful when the lining of the nose has become too dry. Salinex can help to clear excess mucus.

IMMUNOTHERAPY — ARM YOURSELF!

Immunotherapy, also known as 'allergy shots,' 'desensitization' or 'hyposensitization' is a treatment for allergies to pollen, house dust mites and mold. Patients are given gradually increasing doses of the allergen or allergens to which they are sensitive until they reach a maintenance dose. As for timing of shots, injections like those for pollens may be given before the actual season and others year-round for about three to five years, as long as there's evidence an allergic person is improving each year. Keep in mind that allergy shots are not a cure and can't offer complete protection from an allergy. Newer forms of immunotherapy are currently being investigated.

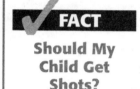

FACT

Should My Child Get Shots?

Allergy shots in patients with allergic rhinitis should only be considered when your child fails environmental control (avoidance) measures and medication is not effective. They are indicated in less than 10 percent of patients with allergic rhinitis.

Comfort Tips

Your child might find relief by using the following remedies:

Drink clear fluids: water, juices and soups keep a child well hydrated.

Use saline nose sprays: help clear excess mucus and humidify the nasal lining.

Humidify a room: keep humidity levels throughout the home at 30 to 50 percent. While running a cold-mist vaporizer or steamy shower may humidify a room, they're not recommended because they can cause excess moisture buildup and be just as harmful as a dry room.

Chapter

4

SKIN CONDITIONS

Eczema (Atopic Dermatitis);
Contact Dermatitis;
Hives (Urticaria);
Skin Swelling (Angioedema)

IN MANY CASES, IT'S NOT UNUSUAL FOR PARENTS to see a skin rash on their child that went away on its own before determining the cause. When skin is red, bumpy, scaly, itchy or swollen, however, you need to pay attention since it can signify a skin condition caused by an immune system reaction. The immune response is complicated, but in recent years, we've developed a better understanding of it and how it creates the skin changes we call inflammation. Like other atopic disorders, such as asthma and hay fever, these skin conditions can be effectively treated to minimize discomfort and disturbance to daily activities. Such skin diseases, which can take several forms and have a number of causes, include the following:

- *Eczema (atopic dermatitis)* — itchy, red, raised and scaly skin often associated with other allergies

- *Contact dermatitis* — a rash caused by irritants and allergens touching the skin

- *Hives (urticaria)* — welts on the skin that can vary in shape and color, and last for hours, days, months, or even years

- *Angioedema* — severe swelling of the deeper layers of the skin that can be disfiguring and uncomfortable

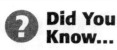 **Did You Know...**

We shed up to 1 gram of dead cells into our bath, clothes and bedding every day. These dead cells provide ready food for dust mites, a common source of allergens.

Your Child's Skin

Before we talk about these skin conditions, you'll want to know a little about the body's skin. Normal, healthy skin acts as a protective barrier between the internal body and the outside world.

Most people think of skin as a thin covering, yet it's the largest organ in the human body.

Human skin has three layers:

1. *Epidermis,* a thin outer protective layer

2. *Dermis,* a middle layer where the blood vessels, nerves, sweat glands and hair roots are located

3. *Inner layer* consisting mainly of insulating fat cells

It's the epidermal and dermal layers that have the most significance to allergists. Epidermal cells are continually being replaced. Old skin cells become flatter and tougher as they age, and eventually die and shed. The mast cells, which are found in the dermal layer among other areas, play an important role — when they come in contact with an allergen, the cells release histamine and other chemicals into the skin to produce an allergic reaction. The skin then becomes inflamed causing redness, swelling and itchiness.

Varying Degrees

◆ ◆ ◆ ◆ ◆

Eczema may look different at various ages. It can range from a scaly rash on most body parts to dry patches in a few areas as she gets older.

WHAT IS ECZEMA?

Eczema (atopic dermatitis) is a common allergic skin disease, which can affect all age groups, but is most common in young children under the age of five. Although the exact cause of eczema is unknown, it's considered a hereditary condition most often associated with food allergies, asthma and/or allergic rhinitis (hay fever). In fact, 80 percent of children with eczema have allergies, yet allergies are only a part of what causes eczema. This skin condition can be very uncomfortable and affect your child's quality of life.

TOP **3** FACTORS IN DIAGNOSING ECZEMA:

1. Skin is extremely itchy

2. Eczematous or bubbly rash

3. An atopic (allergic) individual

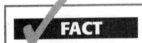

FACT

Eczema's Plight

About 10 percent of infants and children develop eczema. The good news is that eczema tends to improve with age and most children will outgrow the condition.

It Feels and Looks Like...

Almost always, eczema itches. The severity of the disease can vary — in mild forms, the skin is dry, hot and itchy, while in more severe forms, the skin can form cracks, become raw and bleed.

• **In infants**, eczema usually appears as a weepy, scaly rash on the cheeks, scalp, neck, backs of the arms, fronts of the legs or torso. In an attempt to relieve the itching, babies may rub or scratch their faces against a bed sheet or other object and aggravate the eczema by stimulating inflammation.

• **In children and toddlers**, eczema can look like dry, scaly patches usually localized in skin folds, behind the knees, inside the elbows, at the wrists and ankles and at the side of the neck.

• **In teens and adults**, the condition can be limited to one or few areas, such as the hands and feet and around the nipples and lips.

COMMON TRIGGERS

A number of different irritants and allergens can cause flare-ups of eczema. They include:

• **Excessive moisture** from sweating and climate extremes — both cold, dry air and hot, humid weather.

- **Dust mites,** which breed in mattresses and carpeting.

- **Contact with irritants,** such as wool or abrasive fabrics, soaps or detergents.

- **Certain foods.** Food allergy alone is not a common cause of eczema, even when a positive skin test reveals an allergy to a specific food. Your child's doctor may require a food challenge test to confirm the relationship. (See *Chapter 1: Introduction to Allergies* for more information on the test.)

ALLERGY LINK?

There seems to be a connection between eczema and other allergic conditions, and vice versa. Children who have had significant eczema in infancy often develop a sensitivity to airborne allergens (such as dust or molds) at about age two or three years old, whether the eczema is still present or not. However, it's still not clear whether airborne allergens play a role in aggravating eczema. Research shows that about 80 percent of children with severe eczema are at risk of developing asthma or hay fever, while 60 percent of children with troublesome asthma experience eczema at some time.

TREATMENT: STOP THE ITCH

Severe itching is eczema's hallmark and it creates a vicious cycle — your child frequently scratches because of the itch, which tends to aggravate the eczema and worsen the condition. The most effective treatment, then, is to help relieve the itching with some common remedies:

Can I 'Catch' Eczema?

◆ ◆ ◆ ◆ ◆

Eczema can sometimes look unpleasant, with patches that are very dry or ooze clear fluid. But eczema is not contagious, even when you touch it.

Lubricants. The use of bath oils for bathing and the application of emollients after bathing while the skin is still wet can help to relieve dry skin. Use only mild, non-irritating soaps.

Topical corticosteroids. These are applied directly to the skin to reduce the inflammation and control the itch. For example, hydrocortisone cream or ointment is used for mild eczema. More potent, prescription corticosteroids, such as betamethasone and several others, are used when the inflammation is more severe. Only milder forms of topical corticosteroids should be used on the face. Although these medications are safe, overuse can be dangerous. Follow up regularly with your child's physician.

Immunologic or anti-inflammatory therapies. These are a new class of medications that are corticosteroid-free. For example, tacrolimus and picrolimus have been very effective in reducing eczema symptoms, including inflammation and itch.

Oral antihistamines. They can be used to block the histamine effect, which can cause the itching. Aside from minimizing the itch, antihistamines may also have a sedation effect, which will help settle the child. In most cases, they're not sufficient treatment medications on their own and need to be used in conjunction with other treatments.

Oral or local antibiotics. These may be required if the scratching causes a secondary skin infection. Some infections can be quite serious and require more specialized treatments. All infections should be evaluated by your child's physician.

Tar ointments. Dermatologists usually use this therapy in extremely severe cases. Rarely used,

---

Finding a Cure

◆ ◆ ◆ ◆ ◆

There is no cure for eczema. But it can be controlled effectively with medication that decreases the inflammation in the skin.

these ointments can be effective because they soothe inflamed skin. They can be smelly, but newer preparations have less odor and stain less than past formulations.

Phototherapy. Also a rare treatment, UV light waves are used on patients with severe eczema.

7 WAYS TO MANAGE YOUR CHILD'S ECZEMA

1. *Control temperature and humidity.* Keep the temperature of your house (or at least the bedrooms) at 18 to 20 degrees Celsius (64 to 68 degrees Fahrenheit) to avoid excessive sweating, and humidity between 30 to 50 percent to avoid dry skin. (Check humidity levels with a hygrometer.)

2. *Protect and moisturize the skin.* Use creams and emollients on your child's skin before going outside into cold weather and at bedtime, even when the rash isn't visible.

3. *Keep fingernails short and clean.* There is less chance of tearing and infecting the skin from scratching. Children may have to wear gloves at night to prevent scratching.

4. *Wear loose-fitting, cotton clothing.* It's much less likely to irritate the skin than wool, silk, polyester, nylon or linen. Cotton garments can also be layered during the winter months for extra warmth.

5. *Use only a small amount of mild soap.* For bathing and washing clothes/bedding, use gentle soaps and detergents free of perfume or fragrances. Avoid fabric softeners and bleaches, and double rinse thoroughly.

> **? Did You Know...**
>
> Even if you do follow all your doctor's instructions carefully, there may be times when the eczema flares up for no apparent reason. Using a corticosteroid ointment at these times will help relieve the inflammation.

Environment Fix

◆ ◆ ◆ ◆ ◆

Practice environmental control measures to avoid or minimize allergens, such as dust mites, and irritants to the skin, such as direct contact with wool. (See *Chapter 11: Environmental Control* for tips.)

6. ***Bathe daily.*** However, keep the soaking time limited to 10 minutes and use warm, not hot, water. Add about a half to one capful of gentle bath oil to the bathwater during the middle of the bath and use only mild soaps if necessary. After bathing, pat your child dry leaving the skin slightly damp; then apply corticosteroid ointment in specific areas, if needed, and also apply a nonallergenic moisturizer or lubricant — even the areas where the corticosteroid ointment has been applied — in order to protect the skin from becoming too dry.

7. ***Wash off residue of irritating foods.*** Clean your child's face right after eating such foods as strawberries, oranges and tomatoes, therefore reducing the possibility of forming rashes from contact with these foods. Children with such rashes usually have negative skin tests and are not at risk for more severe reactions with such foods.

WHAT IS CONTACT DERMATITIS?

Contact dermatitis is a rash, which can mimic eczema, caused when the skin comes into contact with external agents, such as a certain plant or chemical. Such reactions can be caused when the skin touches an allergen, resulting in an allergic reaction that involves the immune system. Many rashes, however, are caused by nonallergenic or irritant reactions. It can be difficult to tell the difference between a rash caused by an irritant or allergen.

There are two types of contact dermatitis reactions:

Irritant contact dermatitis is a reaction in which the offending substances can damage the skin. The longer the skin is in contact — or the more concentrated the agents — the more severe the reaction. Common irritants include soaps and detergents, so hands are mostly affected.

Allergic contact dermatitis is an itchy, red, blistered reaction that can occur 24 to 48 hours after contact with an allergen. The reaction usually disappears within two to four weeks, even without treatment.

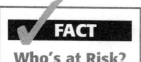

FACT

Who's at Risk?

Contact dermatitis is rare in children and most often occurs in middle-aged and elderly persons. A history of personal or family allergies is not a risk factor.

Affected Body Parts

Different areas of the skin are more sensitive to irritants and allergens than others. The eyelids, neck and genitalia are among the most sensitive, whereas the palms, soles and scalp are more resistant to rash.

COMMON CAUSES OF ALLERGIC CONTACT DERMATITIS

- The poison ivy plant
- Resins from oak and sumac leaves
- Nickel
- Perfumes and fragrances found in soaps, lotions, detergents
- Dyes
- Latex rubber
- Some ingredients in topical medication, such as neomycin, applied directly to the skin

COMMON CAUSES OF IRRITANT CONTACT DERMATITIS

- Soap, cleansing cream, bubble bath, detergents
- Shampoo, conditioner, hair mousse, hairspray
- Shaving cream and after-shave lotion
- Perfume, cosmetic, lipsticks, eye shadow, mascara, nail varnish
- Toothpaste, mouthwash
- Deodorant, depilatory
- Vaginal medication, menstrual pads, tampons
- Athlete's foot lotions, foot powder
- Dye or perfumes in toilet paper
- Nickel in earring studs and other jewellery, lipstick cases, jean studs, button shanks and zippers, coins and key chains
- Plastic rubber in garment waistbands, girdles and socks, stereo headphones, telephone receivers
- Agents used to tan leather for clothing, gloves, shoes, slippers and boots

Finding the Offenders

To determine which agents are causing your child's contact dermatitis, a physician will take an extensive history and conduct an examination. Further testing may involve a series of patches on the back — each contains an extract of the suspecting substance on its surface and is held in place on the skin with reinforcing tape for 48 hours, then the skin is re-examined for any changes.

TREATMENT: SOOTHE THE SKIN

The first course of treatment involves removing or avoiding the irritant or allergen from any contact with the skin. In some cases, the following might also be helpful to relieve an itchy blistered rash:

- Cold water soaks and compresses

- Topical corticosteroids (prescribed if small areas of the skin are affected)

- Oral corticosteroids (prescribed when large areas of the body are involved; which should be continued for the entire duration of the reaction, usually lasting from two to four weeks)

> **? Did You Know...**
>
> It's often very difficult to find an underlying cause for chronic hives. Just the same, your child should see his doctor to rule out any condition, such as an infection, that may be causing the hives.

> ## WHAT ARE HIVES (URTICARIA)?
>
> Hives are actually a type of rash commonly called welts, which can last anywhere from a few hours to days, weeks, months or years at a time. They can appear anywhere on the body and tend to move from one area to another. They can be small or large in diameter, and are usually raised, red lesions that turn white when pressed. They're also frequently itchy.

There are two main types of hives, depending on their duration:

Acute hives are the most common form of urticaria and can occur and disappear spontaneously, lasting minutes or days (usually less than six weeks). Their trigger is often identified, and the most likely causes are:

- A virus, such as the cold or the flu

- Prescribed drugs or over-the-counter preparations, such as vitamins, laxatives, aspirin or herbal remedies

- A certain food, especially a new food or one that is rarely eaten

- Latex rubber products, especially balloons or rubber gloves

- Insect stings

- Exercise

Chronic hives, which last more than six weeks, can occur almost daily for months or years. In about 95 percent of cases, a cause can't be identified. Although food is often thought of as a major cause, it's responsible only in one or two percent of cases.

The persistent nature of chronic hives may sometimes be attributed to an overreaction of the body's immune system. In this case, the body may be reacting against itself such as with certain forms of thyroid disease or arthritis. These particular reactions are more common in adults. In children, viral infections can sometimes initiate chronic hives. The diagnosis, however, isn't always so clear-cut. Because there's often no allergic origin, allergy skin tests are not helpful in identifying the cause of your child's chronic hives. Blood testing may be done to detect a particular disease, but, in children, test results are seldom abnormal.

✔ **FACT**

Hive Dive

Hives usually go away spontaneously or very rapidly with the help of an antihistamine medication.

NONALLERGIC HIVES

There are several specific, nonallergic types of urticaria, caused by a variety of factors. These types include:

- *Dermographism* — hives that develop when the skin is stroked or scratched with a firm object

- *Solar urticaria* — occurs when certain parts of the body are exposed to sunlight

- *Cold-induced urticaria* — appears when exposed to cold temperature, cold water/food or ice. Sometimes the hives appear when the skin is warmed, after exposure to cold

- *Cholinergic (heat-induced) urticaria* — associated with intense exercise, hot showers and/or anxiety

- *Pressure urticaria* — develops from constant pressure from constricting clothing, carrying heavy weights or excessive rubbing of the skin

- *Pregnancy urticaria* — characterized by hives and sometimes swelling, experienced by a number of pregnant women who have never before had an allergy problem

Other causes:

- *X-ray dyes and certain drugs* (aspirin, penicillin and corticosteroids). Drugs cause both allergic and nonallergic hives

- *Infectious diseases* — for example, infectious hepatitis or infectious mononucleosis, fungus or parasite infections and intestinal worms

- *Insect bites* — some of these may come from mosquitoes, bed bugs and fleas

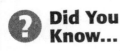

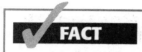

FACT

Hives, Hives Go Away

Chronic hives will clear up in 3 to 12 months in 50 percent of patients; it could take 1 to 5 years for hives to clear up in 40 percent of sufferers; and more than 20 years for their disappearance in 1.5 percent.

TREATMENT: FIND THE CULPRIT

Although the cause of most hives is often uncertain, antihistamines and corticosteroids are often effective in treating them. An allergist may, therefore, prescribe different combinations of these drugs to relieve your child's symptoms until the culprit can be identified and eliminated.

Chronic hives will eventually disappear on their own, with or without treatment, after many weeks or months. But to relieve the itching, an allergist might recommend one or more antihistamines until the best combination is found.

Severe, complicated attacks of hives can be temporarily relieved by adrenaline or antihistamine injections. For acute hives with extensive swelling and breathing difficulties, you should seek emergency medical attention, since injections of adrenaline (epinephrine), antihistamines, corticosteroids and other life-saving measures may be required. In all cases, if possible, the best course of treatment is avoiding the substance that triggers urticaria.

WHAT IS ANGIOEDEMA?

Angioedema is swelling of the deeper layers of the skin, and can sometimes occur with hives. Although the condition is temporary, angioedema can be uncomfortable and disfiguring.

UNDERSTANDING ANGIOEDEMA — Q & A

Q: What does angioedema look like?

A: Angioedema is not red or itchy, and most often occurs in soft tissue, such as in the face, eyelids, mouth/lips or genitals, or on the tongue and in the hands or feet. It may be painful or cause burning. If the swelling is in the throat, it can interfere with breathing and may be life-threatening.

Q: Does angioedema always show up with hives?

A: Often times, angioedema and hives go together, but it can also occur on its own. Both, however, occur when the body releases histamine and other chemicals that are usually stored in mast cells.

Q: How long does angiodema last?

A: Angioedema, like hives, can be acute or chronic. Acute angioedema lasts only a short time (minutes to days) and does not re-occur. Similar triggers responsible for acute urticaria cause it. The chronic type keeps coming back over a long period, and most often, like chronic hives, does not have an obvious cause.

Q: Are there any other forms of angioedema?

A: There is also a rare form of angioedema, which is an inherited disorder (C-1 esterase inhibitor deficiency). It typically involves the lips and tongue and sometimes the throat and stomach. The swelling may be related to trauma in the mouth, such as from dental work. A blood test may help to diagnose this condition. While there is currently no known cure, special medications can reduce the swelling and frequency of attacks.

Chapter

5

ADVERSE FOOD REACTIONS

Allergic and Nonallergic Reactions to Foods

TRUE FOOD ALLERGIES ARE NOT AS COMMON AS you may think, even though about one-quarter of North American households alter their diets because they believe a family member has food allergies. In a recent study of newborns followed until age three, parents reported 28 percent of their children have adversely reacted to a food. However, only eight percent of the reactions could be confirmed by food challenge tests (see "6 Steps to Making a Diagnosis" on page 98 for more details). Because food is an integral part of our lives, it's not surprising that it would be implicated as the cause of many illnesses.

WHAT IS A FOOD ALLERGY?

Most true food allergies or hypersensitivities occur immediately or soon after eating a specific food — within seconds, minutes or a few hours of being ingested. The reaction recurs each time the food is eaten. In this case, the immune system responds to a food protein that the body identifies as foreign. Some reactions that are delayed by a few hours may still be allergic reactions.

What is NOT a Food Allergy?

There are other reactions that happen in the body — while parents label all of them as allergic, doctors refer to them as adverse or abnormal reactions to foods. In these situations, skin testing will produce negative results to a food allergy because the food may be causing a problem through a different mechanism. Some of these reactions might include: toxic reactions, food intolerances or other immune reactions that are not related to allergies.

Allergy Vs. Toxic Vs. Intolerance

Much of the misunderstanding surrounding food allergies has to do with the terms we use to classify them. While food allergies and intolerances can have similar symptoms, their causes and treatments differ. Here's a guide on what these terms really mean:

ADVERSE FOOD REACTIONS

Adverse food reations are any unwanted reactions after ingesting a food or food additive. They include toxic and nontoxic reactions.

- *Toxic food reactions* can happen when you eat enough of a contaminated food. Vomiting and diarrhea, for example, are common reactions after eating food spoiled with salmonella toxins. This is often referred to as food poisoning.

- *Nontoxic reactions* depend on an individual's response to an ingested food. When these reactions are regulated by the immune system, they're known as a food allergy or food hypersensitivity; when they're not regulated by the immune system, they're considered a food intolerance. There are a few exceptions: some immune disorders are unrelated to allergies, such as Celiac disease.

  Food intolerances are dose-specific, meaning that a person may be able to tolerate small servings of a specific food, but experience symptoms when eating larger servings. For example, children with a lactose intolerance lack the enzyme lactase, which helps digest or break down the sugar in milk (lactose) and certain milk products. This enzyme deficiency is common in certain ethnic

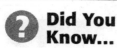 **Did You Know...**

Food allergies in adults are much less common than most people believe, with only 1 to 2 percent of individuals affected and 3 to 4 percent of children.

groups, particularly in Asians. A person with a lactose intolerance may experience bloating, vomiting and diarrhea after drinking a glass of milk, however, he may be able to tolerate smaller amounts of milk. Children with lactose intolerance can also drink special lactose-free milk, which has predigested or broken down sugar.

Adverse Reactions

These reactions include the following breakdowns:

Toxic Reactions	Nontoxic Reactions	
	Immune	*Nonimmune*
• Food poisoning	• Allergic	• Intolerances
	• Nonallergic (Celiac)	

Tiny Nibbles

◆ ◆ ◆ ◆ ◆

Children with a food allergy may react to even small amounts of the suspect food. For example, if they're allergic to milk, even breads that contain milk proteins may cause a reaction.

FOOD FIGHTS

Although our diets consist of a variety of foods, only a few cause the majority of food allergies. These foods will vary in different countries and cultures, depending on whether they're introduced during infancy. For example, in Israel, sesame seed allergy is common during infancy because sesame paste is given to infants like peanut butter is given to North American infants.

The following foods trigger 95 percent of hypersensitivity reactions in North American children:

- Egg
- Peanut
- Milk
- Wheat
- Soy
- Fish

The following foods trigger about 85 percent of North American adolescents' and adults' reactions:

- Peanuts
- Fish
- Shellfish
- Tree nuts

Tree Nuts

If your child is allergic to tree nuts, she'll need to stay away from all nuts. Some of the more common ones in North America include:

- Almonds
- Brazil nuts
- Cashews
- Hazelnuts (filberts)
- Macadamia nuts
- Pecans
- Pine nuts
- Pistachios
- Walnuts

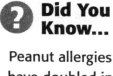

Did You Know...

Peanut allergies have doubled in North America in the last decade, with 1 in 100 North American children now being diagnosed with the allergy. According to researchers, that's because we're being exposed to more peanuts in our food supply.

MULTIPLE WHAMMY?

Multiple food allergies are rare. A study at Johns Hopkins Medical School, which included people who had definite food allergies, revealed that 70 percent had difficulty with just one or two foods, 19 percent reacted to three foods and only three percent reacted to four or more different foods.

4 Most Common Reactions

Like other allergies, the symptoms of food allergies can appear in different ways. They most commonly affect the skin, gastrointestinal tract (bowels), and upper and lower respiratory tracts (throat and lungs) and can range from a few hives to a life-threatening reaction.

1. SKIN

Hives and swelling will usually occur around the eyes, face, lips, hands, feet and genitals. Hives can form around the mouth from simply coming into contact with the food, or they can be scattered all over the body. Hives, which are red, itchy, raised welts, last only a few hours and may change from one part of the body to another. Chronic hives (lasting intermittently for more than six weeks) are rarely caused by a food allergy.

2. GASTROINTESTINAL AREA

These symptoms include stomach cramps, nausea, vomiting, diarrhea and excess gas. They can occur alone or in combination with symptoms from other organ systems.

There are other reactions known as enteropathies that have no connection to allergies, but may occur from milk or soy in the diet. When the stomach and intestines are affected, they'll respond in certain ways, such as with vomiting, diarrhea and abdominal pain, so it's not always easy to tell these disorders apart from allergic conditions. What makes a diagnosis even more difficult is that patients will respond to milk or soy elimination from their diet; however, when patients are tested for a possible allergy, skin tests will show a negative result because there is no allergy to milk or soy. For example, patients with Celiac disease will have a reaction to gluten even though they're not allergic to it.

Tender Tummies

Stomach upsets may not always be related to the food your child is eating. And even when it is, the reaction may not always be associated with a food allergy.

Minimal Risk

◆ ◆ ◆ ◆ ◆

Only about 2 percent of people with food-pollen allergy syndrome or oral allergy syndrome (a type of allergy with symptoms associated with the mouth and throat) are at risk of experiencing a life-threatening anaphylactic reaction.

When allergy tests are negative and your child doesn't respond to eliminating foods from his diet, there are many other gastrointestinal disorders that your doctor may have to consider that are not related to specific food allergies. The list of causes is long — some might include different disorders, such as those that interfere with the absorption of foods (malabsorption syndromes). Your child will need to be evaluated by a gastroenterologist to help sort through these disorders.

What is Food-pollen Allergy Syndrome?

The condition is common in those with sensitivities to trees pollens, particularly birch trees, ragweed and grass. When these people eat certain fresh fruits, vegetables or nuts, they experience itching, burning, tingling and swelling on their lips, inside their mouth and throat. That's because the proteins in these foods are similar to the ones found in plants causing the allergies. The reaction is uncomfortable, but not severe in most cases, and it rarely happens with cooked and canned fruits or vegetables. In rare situations, if the food is completely swallowed, there is a two percent chance of an anaphylactic reaction. This is why people are advised to spit out the food and rinse their mouths immediately to get rid of the offending food.

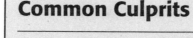

Common Culprits

The most common foods that cause food-pollen allergy syndrome are:

- Apple
- Banana
- Carrot
- Celery
- Hazelnut

- Kiwi
- Melons
- Potato
- Tomato

What is Celiac Disease?

◆ ◆ ◆ ◆ ◆

People with Celiac disease, a type of food intolerance, have a problem breaking down the protein (gluten) in wheat and some other grains. This disease is probably due to an immune response to gluten, but is not an allergic immune response.

---

3. RESPIRATORY TRACT (Nose, throat and chest)

Symptoms such as breathing difficulties, cough, sneezing, wheezing, nose itching and discharge rarely occur on their own after eating a food and are usually part of a generalized anaphylactic (life-threatening) reaction. Respiratory problems alone are rarely caused by food.

4. ANAPHYLAXIS

This refers to a life-threatening reaction that occurs within seconds, minutes or a couple of hours after ingesting a food to which an individual is allergic. Such reactions usually involve hives, swelling, some degree of breathing obstruction and/or a drop in blood pressure, which may cause collapse or even death. (See *Chapter 6: Anaphylaxis* for more details.)

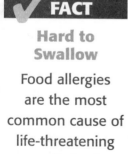

Unusual Suspect

In very rare cases, a child could get exercise-induced anaphylaxis if she exercises within two to four hours of eating a particular food that ordinarily causes no problem. She'll develop hives and breathing difficulties that can be life threatening. Typical suspect foods include: wheat, shellfish, celery and fish. Although rare, it can happen after any meal.

Diagnosis: Does My Child Have a Food Allergy?

Sometimes it's easy for your child's allergist to diagnose a food allergy. For example, if a child's lips and face swell within minutes of eating peanuts, it's obvious that peanuts are the cause of an allergy. Other cases can be more difficult, especially if the offending food is used as an ingredient in many dishes such as the ones you'll find in restaurants.

A common problem in diagnosing food allergies is that people tend to ignore foods as the cause of an allergy if it has been eaten a few times in the past without a reaction. These few exposures may sensitize (make one allergic) to that particular food and the next time the food is eaten, the allergic reaction may occur.

If your child eats a food daily over many years, such as milk, she builds a tolerance and not a sensitization to that food. Therefore, it's highly unlikely, for example, for a 10-year-old who has ingested milk all of his life to suddenly develop a milk allergy.

Top 7 Questions You'll Need to Answer

1. What is the suspect food?

2. How much of the food was eaten?

3. What symptoms did eating the food cause?

4. How long after eating the food did the symptoms begin?

5. Did ingesting the suspected food produce similar symptoms on other occasions?

6. What is the length of time since the last reaction?

7. Are the reactions associated with exercise?

6 STEPS TO MAKING A DIAGNOSIS

Step 1: Keep a **food diary** if your child's medical history doesn't point to the potential culprit. In the diary, list all the foods eaten at each meal, how the foods were prepared and the nature and times of the onset of symptoms. You may see a pattern after reviewing your notes.

Playing It Safe

◆ ◆ ◆ ◆ ◆

Whenever possible, allow your child to eat only home-prepared foods, which are safer.

Step 2: A **physical examination** of the child can be helpful if he shows physical features of other allergic disorders. Many people with food allergies may show signs of other types of allergies, such as eczema, wheezing, or problems with hay fever, such as a congested runny nose and dark circles under the eyes. If the child appears malnourished, it could indicate that he has been on a restricted diet for too long or has some other medical problem.

Step 3: A **skin prick test** will be used by your child's doctor to confirm his suspicions. (See *Chapter 1: Introduction to Allergies* for more information on the skin test.) If the skin test is negative, most patients will usually be able to tolerate the particular food without a reaction. Only a small number of patients with negative skin tests have reactions to a food, making a negative skin test highly reliable. However, a positive skin test is not always as helpful in determining the cause. Therefore, the results of your child's skin tests need to be interpreted by an allergy specialist to help determine the validity of the positive food skin test. For example, if an obvious reaction, such as hives, appears within minutes of eating peanuts and the skin test to peanut is positive, then the diagnosis of a peanut allergy is confirmed. However, if the history is unclear and the child develops a reaction after eating a mixture, then a positive skin test may not be as helpful. Your child's physician may need to do an oral challenge under controlled conditions in order to be certain that peanut or something else was the cause.

Step 4: **RAST/ImmunoCap** is a blood test that is performed when the skin test can't be done (see "Testing, Testing"). However, it's not used to replace the skin test on a routine basis. People assume that because the RAST is done through the blood, it's accurate, but studies show that a properly performed skin test is still the superior test.

The ImmunoCap is a newer version of the RAST and is used in the same circumstances as the RAST. It may be useful, however, in determining if a patient has IgE antibodies (which signify the body's response to an allergen) to specific foods. Depending on the IgE level, the doctor may be able to determine if the patient can safely undergo

---

Testing, Testing

♦ ♦ ♦ ♦ ♦

Skin testing may not be appropriate in all cases. For example, if the patient has severe eczema or is taking medication that could interfere with the testing (for example, antihistamines), it could be difficult to perform the test and get accurate results.

a supervised oral food challenge (see step 6). However, the benefits of this blood test are still being studied, so your doctor may or may not recommend it.

Step 5: Elimination diet is used when the answer is still not obvious. Your child's physician might recommend eliminating one or two suspicious foods from her diet for two weeks and monitoring the reaction. The eliminated foods are then slowly re-introduced and you'll be asked to watch for any symptoms in your child that could be caused when certain foods are eaten.

Step 6: Oral food challenge testing is the most reliable method of confirming a food allergy. The test must be done under a doctor's supervision in his office or, in some cases, in the hospital, where treatment can be given immediately if there is a serious reaction.

Reading Food Labels

The only safe way to prevent a food allergy reaction is to strictly avoid the food that causes problems. It's easy to do if your child is allergic to kiwi or shrimp, but if she's allergic to a basic food, such as milk or egg, which is commonly used as an ingredient in recipes or other packaged foods, it can be more challenging. You may need help from a qualified dietitian to find alternatives and plan a nutritionally balanced diet.

Every member of the family should learn how to read a food label to identify whether a product contains a restricted food. But it can be difficult because there are numerous variations of an ingredient's name. See "How To Read a Label" on page 111 for a detailed list of food protein alternatives and the foods that contain them.

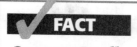

FACT

Can you *Really* Avoid Peanuts?

Studies have found that about 35 to 40 percent of patients allergic to peanuts will experience an accidental peanut ingestion within 3 to 4 years.

How Many Peanuts?

The label "may contain peanut" or "made on shared equipment" doesn't tell consumers how much peanut, if any, is actually in the packaged food. Although most peanut-sensitive individuals will be able to tolerate these products, it's recommended they strictly avoid all foods with this labeling.

Allergy-Free?

◆ ◆ ◆ ◆ ◆

Don't rely on the bold labels on the front of packaged foods for a guide on allergy-free contents. Some labels may state the packaged good is "free" of an ingredient, but that doesn't mean it's free of possible substitutes.

HIDDEN DANGERS

Parents should beware that prepared foods may contain not only the food but various components of the food that causes a child's allergic reaction. Be prepared to read obvious and not-so-obvious components on labels. These alternative names indicate the presence of various foods, such as milk, egg, peanut or nut proteins in prepared foods.

SAFETY FIRST

Even when you're extra cautious, your child can accidentally ingest certain off-limits foods. Practice and enforce these safety procedures when your child gathers for school or recreational activities. (See helpful charts at the back of this chapter starting on page 111.)

✓ Tell friends, schoolmates and relatives about your child's life-threatening food allergies.

✓ Ensure your child wears a MedicAlert bracelet and carries an injectable epinephrine (adrenaline) device at all times if she has a life-threatening allergy. (See *Chapter 10: Coping With Allergies* for more information on using an epinephrine device.) Your child and his caregivers should be taught about the signs and symptoms to look for during an allergic food reaction.

✓ Give your child's school a written emergency action plan, describing the allergy, possible symptoms, medications to be given and emergency phone numbers to call.

ALLERGY AWARE

Dining out with your allergic child doesn't have to be risky. Many restaurants, especially the larger chains, are aware of the public's allergy concerns and have programs in place that can help customers identify ingredient information on their menus. Ask the restaurant's manager about particular programs.

Short Order

◆ ◆ ◆ ◆ ◆

When you and your child eat out at restaurants, ask your food handler/server about the ingredients in a dish. And don't forget to ask about the ingredients in foods at parties.

Read the Label Every Time!

Just because your child has eaten a packaged food before without incidence doesn't mean you should trust its contents every time. Food manufacturers may change the ingredients in their products. Parents should also beware of a "new and improved" sign on the package.

Gastrointestinal Barrier

The reason for developing allergies is unknown. One theory suggests that in the first few months of life, infants are particularly susceptible to developing food allergies because they have what is sometimes described as a 'leaky' or 'open' digestive tract. The mucosal barrier that lines the intestine is immature; it sometimes allows large intact proteins to enter the bloodstream before they are broken down and cause allergic reactions. As the gut matures, the proteins are broken down into smaller components called amino acids, which are less likely to cause food allergies.

Crossing Allergies

◆ ◆ ◆ ◆ ◆

Cross-reactivity within food families is very rare. People who have a severe life-threatening allergy to peanuts (which is part of the legume family) have the same chance as anyone else of developing an allergy to other legumes.

Breast-feeding Benefits

If very young infants develop allergies, it's usually to milk protein in formulas but rarely to breast milk. Breast milk seems to offer some protection against developing allergies, in part, possibly, because of some of its natural ingredients. This is one of the reasons that breast milk, in addition to having many other health benefits, is recommended as the main food source during the first six months of an infant's life.

Breast-fed infants may have better protection over formula-fed babies, but may still develop allergies. One theory is that some allergens from the mother's diet (for example, egg, milk or peanut) cross into her milk. Breast-feeding alone for six months may be able to delay, but not necessarily prevent, her baby from developing eczema. Still, despite these precautions, a child may develop allergies to one of these specific foods later in life. Before starting any restrictive diet, mothers should talk to their family doctor or a professional dietitian.

Formula Feeds

For mothers who are unable to breast-feed, there are a number of formulas available. Some of the specialized formulas can be used for treatment of milk allergies. However, the use of these formulas for the prevention of milk allergies is controversial.

Casein-based or whey-based hydrolysate formulas have their proteins broken down (hydrolyzed) into smaller units and are less of an allergy concern. It has been suggested that these be used for the prevention of allergy. (See *Chapter 12: Prevention of Allergies* for a more detailed explanation of these formulas.) These hydrolyzed formulas can also be used to treat an infant with a milk allergy who may also be allergic to soy.

Soy-based formulas use the proteins from soybeans rather than those found in cow's milk. They can be used as a substitute if the child has a milk allergy and the physician has verified that there is no associated soy allergy. Soy is not effective for the prevention of milk allergies.

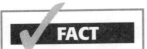 **FACT**

Safe Soy?

There is only a 4 to 7 percent chance that infants with an allergy to cow's-milk protein will also have an allergic reaction to soy.

Goodbye Allergy

Toddlers tend to lose their food allergies to milk and egg. With milk, 50 percent will lose the allergy by the time they are one year old, 70 percent by age two, and 85 percent by age three. An egg allergy is lost in 80 percent of cases between ages three and five years. Peanut is not lost as easily — only 20 percent tend to lose it by five years of age and it's usually only those who've had milder reactions. There is no data for fish. Food allergies, therefore, need to be reassessed every one to two years.

Pregnancy Pitfalls

Some research suggests that allergies in infants can occur before birth, as early as pregnancy. When the risk of allergy is high, some doctors may recommend placing mothers on special diets during the last three months (or even earlier) of pregnancy. However, because there is little scientific evidence to date to support this move, physicians rarely recommend restrictions, which can jeopardize the nutritional status of the mother and her fetus.

Introducing Solids

When Can My Child Eat...?

◆ ◆ ◆ ◆ ◆

In North America, it's recommended that parents introduce foods commonly causing reactions at certain ages. However, this is not recommended in Europe. See *Chapter 12: Prevention of Allergies* for more details.

Some studies have shown that not adding any solids before six months of age may help prevent the development of allergies. (See *Chapter 12: Prevention of Allergies* for more information.) It's recommended that parents introduce new foods to their babies one at a time in order to better track any adverse reactions. Here's how:

● Initially, introduce foods as single ingredients. That means you start with single-grain infant cereals, such as rice cereal, before introducing your infant to a cereal that is a mixture of several grains or fruit. Take a week to work up to a full serving.

● If you notice a reaction, such as spitting up or diarrhea after first introducing a new food, stop feeding it to your baby but try it again in very small amounts a few weeks later, once all the symptoms have cleared. Don't assume that your baby is automatically allergic to the specific food. If you observe the same symptoms twice, discuss them with your doctor.

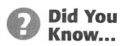 **Did You Know...**

While food additives have been blamed for a wide range of adverse reactions, from mood and behavior changes to severe asthma and anaphylaxis, allergic reactions to food additives are very rare. In a British study, 7 percent of respondents thought they had a sensitivity to food additives. However, in a follow-up challenge test, only 3 people, or less than 0.25 percent, had true symptoms to an additive allergy.

- There's a difference of opinion on when to add certain highly allergenic foods. In high-risk families where there is a history of food allergies, North American researchers recommend you introduce cow's milk to your child at one year, egg at two years, peanut and fish at three years. The Europeans feel there is no evidence for this approach and add these foods at any time after the first five months of age. It's not necessary to avoid foods before certain ages in order to prevent allergies in families where there is no evidence of any allergic problems.

The Scoop on Solids

A baby with a family history of allergies should be given only one new food a week, starting with one small teaspoon. If there are no problems, you can increase the serving size over the next week until your baby is receiving a full normal serving. Adding foods in this manner could help you detect when small amounts of food are causing an allergic reaction in your child, so that you can stop adding it into your child's diet before a larger amount possibly brings out the allergy.

Food Additives

Many substances are added to food to enhance its texture, color or flavor, or to prevent it from spoiling. Such food additives can be divided into a number of categories, depending on their purpose.

However, the more common ones associated with adverse reactions fall into the following four categories:

1. Food coloring agents
2. Preservatives
3. Flavor enhancers
4. Sweeteners

1. FOOD COLORING

Food colorants can be either synthetic or natural. The synthetic dye tartrazine has been implicated in causing adverse reactions, such as asthma symptoms and hives, although no studies have ever proven this. You'll find the colorant in cake and icing mixes, puddings, pie fillings, ice creams, drink mixes and soft drinks.

Adverse Additives?

◆ ◆ ◆ ◆ ◆

While some allergic reactions to food additives have been reported, more research is needed to confirm a link.

Common Colorants

Here are some of the more common ones you'll read on food labels.

Synthetic dyes in foods:	Natural colorants in foods:
• Tartrazine (yellow dye #5)	• Annatto
• Sunset yellow (yellow dye #6)	• Carmine
• Amaranth (red dye #2)	• Carotene
• Erythrosine (red dye #3)	• Turmeric
• Ponceau (red dye #4)	• Paprika
• Brilliant blue (blue dye #1)	• Beet extract
• Indigotine (blue dye #2)	• Grape skin extract

Hyperactive Link

In 1973, Dr. Benjamin Feingold wrote a book that claimed tartrazine, other food coloring agents and natural salicylates in foods caused hyperactivity, behavior problems and learning disabilities in children. Parents who were desperate to find a cure for a child's difficult behavior placed them on diets that avoided foods containing these additives. Feingold claimed that 50 percent of hyperactive children improved on such diets, however, many independent studies have never shown a relationship between diet and behavior.

2. PRESERVATIVES

Sulfites. They're used to prevent foods from browning and spoiling. You'll find high concentrations of sulfites in foods such as dried fruits, lemon juice, lime juice, wine, molasses, sauerkraut and grape juice. In a few asthmatics, sulfites can precipitate symptoms ranging from mild wheezing to life-threatening reactions. Sulfites used as food or drug additives include:

Preserving Asthma

◆ ◆ ◆ ◆ ◆

About 5 percent of asthmatics are reported to have asthmatic attacks from sulfites.

- Sulphur dioxide
- Inorganic sulfite salts
- Sodium and potassium metabisulfite
- Sodium and potassium bisulfite
- Sodium sulfites

Sodium benzoate and **benzoic acid.** They're used widely to inhibit the growth of microorganisms in foods such as cereals, cakes and instant potatoes. Benzoic acid also occurs naturally in cranberries, raspberries, prunes and other foods. Several cases of adverse reactions to benzoates have been recorded. Hives, swelling and anaphylactic reactions have previously been reported.

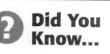

Butylated hydroxyanisole (BHA) and **butylated hydroxytoluene (BHT)** are antioxidants used in cereals and other grain products to maintain crispiness; used in oils, BHA and BHT prevent them from going rancid. There are no well-documented reports of allergic reactions to these preservatives.

Nitrates and **nitrites** are used as curing agents in meat products, for example, salami, ham and bologna. They've been implicated as a cause of chronic hives (chronic urticaria), although this has not been well established, as well as possible triggers of severe headaches.

3. FLAVOR ENHANCERS

Monosodium glutamate (MSG) is one of the most commonly used food additives, but it also occurs naturally in almost all foods. MSG in large quantities has been reported to cause burning of the skin and flushing, chest pressure and tightness, tingling and numbness of the face, neck, upper chest and arms, dizziness, nausea, vomiting and headaches — also known as Chinese Restaurant Syndrome because it was often used in many chinese dishes in the past. More recently, MSG has been linked to triggering asthma, but more studies are needed to prove this association.

4. SWEETENERS

Aspartame is a low-calorie sweetener found in many foods, including fruit juices, gum, breath mints and carbonated drinks. There have been a few reports of hives after ingesting aspartame, but controlled studies have not confirmed hypersensitivity reactions to it.

TAKING A BITE OUT OF ALLERGIES — Q & A

Q: My child is allergic to peanuts. Should he stay away from foods in the same food family?

A: In the past, allergists recommended eliminating all foods from the same family if one member was known to cause allergies. So in your child's case, he was advised to avoid other legumes such as peas. (Note that peanut is a legume, not a nut.) We now know that although cross reactions are possible, they don't necessarily occur within the same food families. Therefore, it's unnecessary to eliminate entire food families and, therefore, not risk jeopardizing a child's nutritional balance.

However, there are cross reactions outside food families and within the plant kingdom in general. Nuts, which fall into several different food families, have a 30 percent chance of crossing over with peanut. Therefore, you need to ask your allergist about food relationships that are important to your child's food allergy.

Q: Will my child have to live with food allergies the rest of his life?

A: Many food allergies diagnosed in infancy are not lifelong. Within a few years, most young children outgrow (or become tolerant of) their food hypersensitivity, except in most cases of peanut, tree nut and seafood allergies. They tend to lose their reactivity to milk, soy, eggs and wheat as they get older. Food allergies begin in infants in the first year of life about 80 percent of the time.

Q: Can certain drugs prevent a food allergy?

A: Drugs have been tested to prevent a food allergy reaction, but the results to date have been disappointing. Various antihistamines, sodium cromoglycate (Intal) and ketotifen (Zaditen) have not been very effective. Research to determine if patients can be desensitized to a peanut allergy by injections (immunotherapy) of small doses of peanut was discontinued because patients were experiencing too many reactions from the treatment. Today, research is focusing on the development of vaccines and on blocking Immunoglobulin E (IgE) antibodies that are responsible for allergy symptoms (anti-IgE therapy). These new methods appear to modify the problem but not completely eliminate the allergy. For example, a recent vaccine tested to suppress peanut allergies boosted a person's tolerance to about nine peanuts with minimal side effects. More research on vaccines is underway. (See *Chapter 12: Prevention of Allergies* for more information about new developments.)

How To Read a Label

Even when you read a food label to determine whether an allergenic food is used to make the product, you can find yourself overwhelmed by all the technical terms. Here, we've included a series of charts to help you decipher which foods contain an allergenic ingredient and the presence of certain food proteins, which can be just as harmful to your child.

How To Read a Label for an EGG-FREE DIET

Avoid foods that contain eggs or any of these ingredients:	May indicate the presence of egg protein:
• Albumin (also spelled as albumen)	• Flavoring (including natural and artificial)
• Egg (dried, powdered, solids, white, yolk)	• Lecithin
• Eggnog	• Macaroni
• Lysozyme	• Marzipan
• Mayonnaise	• Marshmallows
• Meringue (meringue powder)	• Nougat
• Surimi	• Pasta

Chart reprinted with permission from The Food Allergy & Anaphylaxis Network.

How To Read a Label for a MILK-FREE DIET

Avoid foods that contain milk or any of these ingredients

- Artificial butter flavor
- Butter, butter fat, butter oil
- Buttermilk
- Casein (casein hydrolysate)
- Caseinates (in all forms)
- Cheese
- Cream
- Cottage cheese
- Curds
- Custard
- Ghee
- Half & half
- Lactalbumin, lactalbumin phosphate
- Lactoferrin
- Lactulose
- Milk (in all forms including condensed, derivative, dry, evaporated, goat's milk and milk from other animals, low-fat, malted, milkfat, non-fat, powder, protein, skimmed, solids, whole)
- Nougat
- Pudding
- Rennet casein
- Sour cream, sour cream solids
- Sour milk solids
- Whey (in all forms)
- Yogurt

May indicate the presence of milk protein

- Caramel candies
- Chocolate
- Flavorings (including natural and artificial)
- High protein flour
- Lactic acid starter culture
- Lactose
- Luncheon meat, hot dogs, sausages
- Margarine
- Nondairy products

Chart reprinted with permission from The Food Allergy & Anaphylaxis Network.

How To Read a Label for a PEANUT-FREE DIET

Avoid foods that contain peanuts or any of these ingredients

- Artificial nuts
- Beer nuts
- Cold pressed, expelled, or extruded peanut oil
- Goobers
- Ground nuts
- Mandelonas
- Mixed nuts
- Monkey nuts
- Nutmeat
- Nut pieces
- Peanut
- Peanut butter
- Peanut flour

May indicate the presence of peanut protein

- African, Asian (especially Chinese, Indian, Indonesian, Japanese, Thai and Vietnamese), and Mexican dishes
- Baked goods (pastries, cookies, etc.)
- Candy (including chocolate candy)
- Chili
- Egg rolls
- Enchilada sauce
- Flavoring (including natural and artificial)
- Marzipan
- Nougat

- Studies show that most allergic individuals can safely eat peanut oil (*not* cold pressed, expelled, or extruded peanut oil).

- Arachis oil is peanut oil.

- Experts advise patients allergic to peanuts to avoid tree nuts as well.

- A study showed that unlike other legumes, there is a strong possibility of cross reaction between peanuts and lupine.

- Sunflower seeds are often produced on equipment shared with peanuts.

Chart reprinted with permission from The Food Allergy & Anaphylaxis Network.

How To Read a Label for a WHEAT-FREE DIET

Avoid foods that contain wheat or any of these ingredients

- Bran
- Bread crumbs
- Bulgur
- Couscous
- Cracker meal
- Durum
- Farina
- Flour (all-purpose, bread, durum, cake, enriched, graham, high gluten, high protein, instant, pastry, self-rising, soft wheat, steel ground, stone ground, whole wheat)
- Gluten

- Kamut
- Matzoh, matzoh meal (also spelled as matzo)
- Pasta
- Seitan
- Semolina
- Spelt
- Vital gluten
- Wheat (bran, germ, gluten, malt, sprouts)
- Wheat grass
- Whole wheat berries

May indicate the presence of wheat protein

- Flavoring (including natural and artificial)
- Hydrolyzed protein
- Soy sauce

- Starch (gelatinized starch, modified starch, modified food starch, vegetable starch, wheat starch)
- Surimi

Chart reprinted with permission from The Food Allergy & Anaphylaxis Network.

How To Read a Label for a SOY-FREE DIET

Avoid foods that contain soy or any of these ingredients

- Edamame
- Hydrolyzed soy protein
- Miso
- Natto
- Shoyu sauce
- Soy (soy albumin, soy fiber, soy flour, soy grits, soy milk, soy nuts, soy sprouts)
- Soya

- Soybean (curd, granules)
- Soy protein (concentrate, isolate)
- Soy sauce
- Tamari
- Tempeh
- Textured vegetable protein (TVP)
- Tofu

May indicate the presence of soy protein

- Asian cuisine
- Flavoring (including natural and artificial)
- Vegetable broth

- Vegetable gum
- Vegetable starch

- Studies show most individuals allergic to soy may safely eat soy lecithin and soybean oil.

Chart reprinted with permission from The Food Allergy & Anaphylaxis Network.

How To Read a Label for a TREE NUT-FREE DIET

Avoid foods that contain nuts or any of these ingredients

- Almonds
- Artificial nuts
- Brazil nuts
- Caponata
- Cashews
- Chestnuts
- Filbert/hazelnuts
- Gianduja (a nut mixture found in some chocolate)
- Hickory nuts
- Macadamia nuts
- Mandelonas
- Marzipan/almond paste
- Nan-gai nuts
- Natural nut extract (i.e., almond, walnut)

- Nougat
- Nut butters (i.e., cashew butter)
- Nut meal
- Nutmeat
- Nut oil
- Nut paste (i.e., almond paste)
- Nut pieces
- Pecans (Mashuga Nuts)
- Pesto
- Pine nuts (also referred to as Indian, piñon, pinyon, pignoli, pigñolia and pignon nuts)
- Pistachios
- Pralines
- Walnuts

Keep the following in mind:

- Mortadella may contain pistachios.
- Natural and artificial flavoring may contain tree nuts.
- Experts advise patients allergic to tree nuts to avoid peanuts as well.
- Talk to your doctor if you find other nuts not listed here.

Chart reprinted with permission from The Food Allergy & Anaphylaxis Network.

How To Read a Label for a SHELLFISH-FREE DIET

Avoid foods that contain shellfish or any of these ingredients

- Abalone
- Clams (cherrystone, littleneck, pismo, quahog)
- Cockle (periwinkle, sea urchin)
- Crab
- Crawfish (crayfish, ecrevisse)
- Lobster (langouste, langoustine, scampo, coral, tomalley)
- Mollusks

- Mussels
- Octopus
- Oysters
- Prawns
- Scallops
- Shrimp (crevette)
- Snails (escargot)
- Squid (calamari)

May indicate the presence of shellfish protein

- Bouillabaisse
- Cuttlefish ink
- Fish stock
- Flavoring (including natural and artificial)

- Seafood flavoring (such as crab or clam extract)
- Surimi

Keep the following in mind:

- Any food served in a seafood restaurant may be cross contaminated with fish or shellfish.
- For some individuals, a reaction may occur from cooking odors or from handling fish or shellfish.
- Always carry medications and use them as soon as symptoms develop.

Chart reprinted with permission from The Food Allergy & Anaphylaxis Network.

Chapter 6

ANAPHYLAXIS

Severe Allergic Reactions

WHILE ANAPHYLAXIS CAN BE FATAL, NOT all reactions are as severe. Just the same, any child who has experienced a severe reaction affecting many systems of the body such as the skin, cardiovascular, gastrointestinal or respiratory, needs to take precautions. In all instances, it's important for parents to pay particular attention to certain symptoms and be ready to access immediate treatment.

WHAT IS ANAPHYLAXIS?

A serious allergic reaction that affects many parts of the body at once and is potentially **life threatening**. It can occur within minutes or hours of contacting a specific trigger, such as a particular food, insect sting or medication. It can even be caused by latex or strenuous exercise.

Scaling Symptoms

◆ ◆ ◆ ◆ ◆

Symptoms of an allergic reaction can be very mild, such as a few spots on the skin, but may include more severe symptoms, such as anaphylactic shock or seizure.

Know the Warning Signs

It can be frightening for a parent to know that anaphylaxis wears many faces — the symptoms of a reaction can be the same with each episode but can vary from one individual to the next and from one episode to the next. In most cases, a child's symptoms will include multiple areas of the body, such as the skin, stomach, breathing passages, heart and blood vessels. A reaction can be fatal if it's not treated immediately. (See "Treatments" section further in the chapter on page 126.)

Your child may experience these **symptoms** during an anaphylactic reaction:

- Hives. They can range from a few isolated hives to rapidly spreading hives throughout the body. (See *Chapter 4: Skin Conditions* for more information.)

- Swelling of face, lips, tongue or eyes, hands, feet or genitalia

- Persistent coughing, difficulty breathing, wheezing, chest tightness

- Throat tightness, difficulty swallowing or talking

- Rapid or irregular heart rate

- Red, watery eyes

- Runny nose, sneezing

- Itchiness

- Redness or flushing of different parts of the body

- Significant tummy pain, nausea, vomiting, diarrhea

- A sense of fear or impending doom

- Feeling weak, dizzy or faint

- Collapse, seizures, loss of consciousness

ACT EARLY, NOT LATER!

No matter the initial reaction, caregivers must administer treatment at the start of a reaction and not wait to see if it gets worse, since reactions can intensify within minutes for up to two hours. There could be a delayed response or a second reaction up to 24 hours later. Treatment involves administering a rescue drug called epinephrine (adrenaline) at the start of the reaction, then rushing the child to the

---

What's Involved?

◆ ◆ ◆ ◆ ◆

An anaphylactic episode can involve 1 or more of the following areas:

- Skin
- Respiratory
- Gastrointestinal
- Cardiovascular system

local emergency department (see "Treatments" later in the chapter for more information on devices containing epinephrine, such as the EpiPen, and their use). At the hospital, expect your child to be monitored for four hours or longer, depending on the severity of the reaction.

WHAT HAPPENS DURING ANAPHYLAXIS?

During an anaphylactic episode, a specific trigger attacks certain cells in the blood, primarily the mast cell. In the case where the trigger is an allergic-causing substance (allergen), the trigger binds to the defensive structures on the cell surface known as IgE antibodies. The result is the release of certain chemicals, one of which is histamine, producing different symptoms of anaphylaxis in your child.

Deadly Triggers

◆ ◆ ◆ ◆ ◆

The most common allergens that can cause a potentially lethal anaphylactic reaction include:

- Peanuts
- Tree nuts
- Shellfish
- Exercise
- Insect stings
- Certain antibiotics
- Latex rubber

Making a Prediction

No crystal ball can warn parents of future reactions. There are no symptoms from an earlier reaction or specific test that can help predict the next anaphylactic reaction. Any subsequent reaction could be the same, better or worse. For example, about 20 percent of children with mild facial rashes to peanut can have life-threatening reactions the next time they ingest peanuts. For this reason, parents are encouraged to act quickly if a child who has a history of a mild reaction to a trigger develops any future reaction.

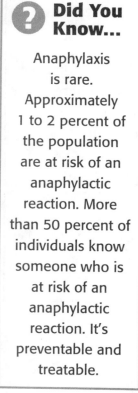

✓ **FACT**

Contaminated Air?

Research shows that the fumes from certain foods, such as peanut butter, do not cause life-threatening reactions. It's only when an offending food is ingested that a reaction will occur.

? **Did You Know...**

Anaphylaxis is rare. Approximately 1 to 2 percent of the population are at risk of an anaphylactic reaction. More than 50 percent of individuals know someone who is at risk of an anaphylactic reaction. It's preventable and treatable.

Who Might Be At Risk?

- *Children with asthma.* One of the theories is that their lungs contain an increased amount of mast cells, that is, the very cells that also are involved in the anaphylactic attacks. These children may have an even greater risk if their asthma is not well controlled.

- *Children with a previous severe anaphylactic attack.* They may be primed because their mast cells are more sensitized.

- *Children with a reaction to peanut, nuts or shellfish.* The reactions to these foods tend to be more severe.

- *Children who take beta-blocker medication.* Beta-blockers (medications used to treat such conditions as heart problems, migraines, tremors), can block the effect of epinephrine, the drug used to treat anaphylactic reactions.

Common Causes

- *Certain foods.* Food is the most common cause, especially peanuts, tree nuts (in North America, the most common ones are walnuts, pecans, pistachios, almonds) and shellfish. Other common foods in North America include milk, egg, wheat, soy, fish and sesame seed. However, almost any food can cause an allergic reaction and go on to be life threatening. Other countries may have different foods that are responsible depending on which foods are more commonly eaten.

- **Insects stings.** Most of these are from stinging insects that belong to the hymenoptera group. They include the yellow jacket, yellow hornet, white-faced hornet, wasp and honeybee. Biting insects don't cause problems to the same extent.

- **Medication.** Although several medications can cause anaphylaxis, the biggest culprits are antibiotics, such as penicillin, especially since they're commonly used to treat bacterial infections in children. Other medications that can cause anaphylaxis include NSAIDS, anti-convulsants, as well as anesthetics.

- **Latex rubber.** A relatively new cause since the regular use of latex rubber gloves in the medical and dental professions about 15 years ago. Contact with moist areas of the body, such as when performing surgery or dental work, poses the greatest risk, while breathing in particles or exposure can also cause a reaction.

- **Exercise.** Strenuous exercise has been linked to some episodes of anaphylaxis. The mechanism for exercise-induced anaphylaxis is not well understood, but is a real risk that requires awareness. Rarely, a child could get exercise-induced anaphylaxis if he exercises within two to four hours of eating a certain food that isn't normally a problem. (See *Chapter 5: Adverse Food Reactions* for more information.)

Get Picky

◆ ◆ ◆ ◆ ◆

If your child has food-related anaphlaxis, ask how food is prepared before letting him taste it when eating out. If you're adding a new product to the grocery cart, read labels carefully. And make sure your child is always carrying epinephrine, which comes in a self-injectable device.

Testing: Making a Diagnosis

In some cases, the diagnosis is obvious when a reaction has occurred immediately after eating a food or receiving an insect sting. But, in other situations, the array of anaphylaxis symptoms can also mimic other conditions, such as fainting spells, anxiety attacks, low blood sugar, asthma or epilepsy. Therefore, it's important to conduct further testing to confirm anaphylaxis or rule out other conditions. If this is the case, your family doctor will refer you to an allergist, who will take a detailed history of the reaction and conduct some tests. If the reaction appears to be caused by an allergen, the allergist may perform skin testing: (For more information on how these tests are performed, see *Chapter 1: Introduction to Allergies.*)

No-no Treatment

Many parents are afraid to give adrenaline injections and opt for an antihistamine. However, antihistamines should not be used as a first-line treatment since they can mask the appearance of more severe symptoms and lead to further problems. The use or non-use of these medications should be discussed on an individual basis with your child's doctor.

Treatments

Epinephrine (adrenaline). Epinephrine is a hormone produced by the body's adrenal glands in response to stressful situations. In drug form, it is the first line of medication used to treat anaphylaxis, but it must be administered soon after the attack starts.

Epinephrine comes in a self-injectable device known as the EpiPen, which is available in two sizes — a junior size for children up to 22 to 25 kilograms (48 to 55 pounds) and an adult size for children above this weight. Physicians recommend giving the EpiPen as soon as a reaction begins. In cases where a child has experienced a previous severe reaction, it's recommended the medication be given *as soon as* there has been contact with a trigger and *before* any reaction begins. Patients should call for an ambulance and have their child transferred to hospital immediately once epinephrine is administered.

Other epinephrine products. There are other pre-loaded syringes, such as the Ana-Kit, which contains two adjustable doses of epinephrine. The syringe devices are more difficult to use and should be discussed with your physician. Inhalers containing epinephrine are also available, however, they can't provide the same protection as the EpiPen because the dose delivered by this route is unreliable. In addition, most children don't like the taste of the inhalation and are unable to take the required number of puffs. Therefore, we can't recommend this device for the treatment of anaphylaxis.

EpiPen Safety

◆ ◆ ◆ ◆ ◆

Once you've used the EpiPen auto-injector, discard it to minimize the chance of injury to others. Ask your doctor or pharmacist about proper disposal methods.

Side Effects

Using epinephrine can cause rapid heart rate, flushing or paleness, dizziness, weakness, tremors and headaches. All these side effects, however, are generally mild and subside in a few minutes. There's only a real concern for individuals with heart disease and high blood pressure — usually limited to adults. Sulfite, which is used as a preservative in syringes, does not cause any problems for individuals with sulfite sensitivity.

Keep Them Posted

◆ ◆ ◆ ◆ ◆

Always provide caregivers with information on your child's allergies. Ensure substitute teachers, volunteers and occasional caregivers also have access to this information.

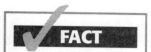

✔ FACT

Read Your Labels

Self-injector devices like the EpiPen have expiry dates of 12 to 18 months after purchase.

Be Prepared: A Guide For Parents

- *Always carry an EpiPen device if you are more than 20 minutes from a medical facility.* Your child may require a second injection 10 to 20 minutes later if the reaction continues or becomes worse. While additional epinephrine (more than two injections) may help, other medications in hospital may be needed at that point to stave off further reaction.

- *If you or your child is traveling with an EpiPen, check with the carrier's policy on carrying one on board.* In most cases, you'll be required to have a signed letter by your child's physician. Also, always be aware of local emergency services and how to access them if needed. Carry a cell phone to access medical attention in emergencies.

- *Get training and help educate caregivers on emergency protocols.* Discuss a child's anaphylactic condition with his teacher and principal and draft an emergency action plan. Make arrangements for storing epinephrine devices at school or, better yet, arrange for your child to carry one if he's responsible enough. For more information about schools and their roles in caring for your child, contact Anaphylaxis Canada (www.anaphylaxis.org) or Canadian Allergy, Asthma and Immunology Foundation (www.allergyfoundation.ca/brochures.html).

- *Recognize the signs and symptoms of a reaction.* Call 911 and tell the operator that a child is having a life-threatening allergic reaction.

- *Avoid long-distance travel where medical help may not be readily available* or a certain trigger, such as insects, may not be avoidable.

- *Ensure your child always wears a MedicAlert bracelet or necklace* to warn others about his allergy problem.

Travel Tips

♦ ♦ ♦ ♦ ♦

To ensure a safe trip with your child, always call the airline ahead of time to alert them about your child's allergic condition. For more tips, see *Chapter 10: Coping with Allergies.*

Minimize the Risk

Here are some main points on staying clear of potentially life-threatening allergens. For further details, see *Chapter 10: Coping With Allergies* and the chapters on the individual causes.

✓ See a qualified allergist for any questions and medical advice about your child's allergies.

✓ Verify the information you've gathered on your child's allergic condition with his family doctor or allergist. Get in contact with reliable sources for current, up-to-date information and research.

✓ Food avoidance — among many challenges, prepare foods at home; avoid unsafe foods such as bulk or imported foods; read labels carefully; take precautions when dining out, eating away from home and handling food; don't trade or share foods or utensils. Ensure your child's school, nursery or day-care center has an allergy-safe program in place.

✓ Insect avoidance — in particular, ensure garbage is stored in a well-covered container and is well clear of playing areas; encourage your child to always use a straw when drinking outside; don't let him walk barefoot in the grass; have him wear light-colored clothing; avoid him from wearing perfume or scented products; keep insecticides readily available.

✓ Drug avoidance — ensure caregivers are aware of specific drugs he's allergic to; become familiar with drugs your child is allergic to; ensure medical personnel are aware of the allergy.

✓ Latex avoidance — become familiar on whether your child falls into a high-risk group; know which products include latex; find alternative products that are latex-free; avoid exposure to environments with latex use.

✓ Wear a MedicAlert identifier.

✓ Know what to do in an emergency, in particular, using the EpiPen.

✓ Educate your child and caregivers about life-threatening allergens and emergency care.

✓ Always be aware, especially when you're away from home, where the nearest hospitals are located and know how to access the local police and ambulance services in the area.

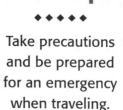

Safe Trip

◆ ◆ ◆ ◆ ◆

Take precautions and be prepared for an emergency when traveling.

? Did You Know...

By using a diary, you can keep track of situations when your child's symptoms have become better or worse.

QUIZ — MYTHS AND MISCONCEPTIONS

This quiz was reprinted with permission from Anaphylaxis Canada, who conducted a study in 2001 to examine deaths from anaphylaxis in the province of Ontario between 1986-2000. The number of deaths investigated was 32.

People rarely die from food-induced anaphylaxis in their own homes.

FALSE.
Thirty out of 32 of the people in this study died in their own homes.

People who experience "mild" reactions to peanuts, tree nuts or shrimp will probably never have a fatal reaction.

FALSE.
Six out of 32 people had experienced "mild" reactions in the past. Five out of 30 had never reported their symptoms to a physician.

Most food-allergic people who die from anaphylaxis are not carrying epinephrine at the time of death because they are noncompliant.

FALSE.
Eleven out of 32 people had been prescribed epinephrine. Four out of 11 had it "close by" at the time of their reaction, but timing of administration was difficult to ascertain. Only one person had refused to carry epinephrine despite a history of severe reactions and another felt that they could not afford it.

Anaphylaxis deaths in restaurants are usually due to cross-contamination.

FALSE.

Trace cross-contamination could possibly have played a role in three out of 32 deaths for which an allergen was not clearly identified.

There have been severe reactions and even deaths on airlines following exposure to peanut dust or trace peanut protein residue on seats.

FALSE.

There was one in-flight death in the study. It followed actual ingestion of food and did not involve either peanut or tree nut.

Simply the smell of peanut butter can trigger a severe or even fatal reaction.

FALSE.

All fatalities followed actual ingestion of food. There were also two examples of a peanut butter-contaminated knife.

The first sign of food allergy is often a fatal allergic reaction.

FALSE.

At least 10 out of 32 people had shown some prior reactivity to their allergen. Two out of six people who died from ingestion of tree nuts knew that they were allergic to peanut but had not been tested for tree nuts.

Chapter 7

INSECT ALLERGIES

Allergies to Insect Stings and Bites

A T SOME POINT IN THEIR LIVES, MOST KIDS WILL experience the unpleasant swelling, redness and pain associated with an insect sting. The vast majority of these reactions will be mild and short-lived. But a few children may experience potentially life-threatening allergic reactions. Unfortunately, insect allergies cannot be predicted, but an allergist can help diagnose whether your child has had an allergic reaction and provide treatment and preventive measures.

Mystery Reaction

◆ ◆ ◆ ◆ ◆

Many patients have had multiple uneventful stings before experiencing their first allergic reaction, while others experience anaphylaxis with their first sting. Unfortunately, allergists can't predict these reactions.

WHAT IS AN INSECT ALLERGY?

Allergic reactions to insect bites and stings occur when the affected child's immune system produces IgE antibodies to the venoms produced by the insect. The IgE antibodies force the release of histamine and other chemicals the next time the person is stung. These chemicals cause hives, swelling, and/or more severe symptoms. Why do some kids produce the antibodies — and develop the associated allergic response — and not others? No one knows for sure.

Normal Reactions

Almost everyone reacts to the irritants and toxins found in the saliva of biting insects and in the venom of stinging insects. It's normal and doctors refer to this normal response as a localized reaction. So what does normal look like? You can expect your child to display the following symptoms:

- Mild redness and swelling at the involved site. This reaction usually occurs within a few minutes and disappears within several hours.

- Severe swellings and redness extending from the area of the bite or sting. Although alarming in appearance, this is usually treated the same way as a normal reaction. It often continues to grow for 24 to 48 hours and may last up to seven to 10 days. Extra medications may be required for such prolonged reactions.

- Fatigue, nausea and malaise may be part of a reaction.

- Bites or stings around the face, eyes and neck often become much larger because the skin in these areas is quite loose.

- Insect bites and stings can become infected if scratched. Infected sites will appear red, raw and may secrete fluid. (Swelling that occurs within the first 24 to 48 hours is normal and is not due to infection.) Only about 10 percent of children will experience infection.

Allergic Reactions

So, what if your child's reaction looks anything but normal? Then you may be dealing with an allergy. Only about three percent of children will suffer from insect allergies, with adults slightly more prone to the allergic response.

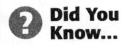 **Did You Know...**

Approximately 50 people die of insect stings in the United States each year, although there may be a few unrecognized fatalities because the sting may not have been witnessed.

Allergic reactions are called generalized reactions because they usually involve areas of the body — most often the skin, throat, lungs, heart and digestive system — away from the site of the bite or sting. When these reactions become life threatening, they are referred to as anaphylaxis. (See *Chapter 6: Anaphylaxis* for more information and emergency treatment.)

You'll know your child is having an anaphylactic response if you see him exhibiting the following symptoms:

- Swelling or hives over the body and face

- Swelling of the tongue and larynx (voice box). Swelling in the throat can produce hoarseness or difficulty swallowing

- Difficulty breathing, wheezing

- Nausea, vomiting, diarrhea and abdominal pain

- Light-headedness, rapid heartbeat, feelings of impending doom, profuse sweating, loss of consciousness or convulsion

If your child displays any of these symptoms, she may be in danger of anaphylaxis. Seek immediate medical attention.

✔ **FACT**

Soothing the Sting

Studies show that less than 5 percent of adults and children who suffer localized responses to an insect sting will go on to have a more serious reaction with the next sting.

Severe Reaction Risk

In rare cases, other reactions — including hives, joint pain, malaise and fever — may occur one week after an insect sting. Children with such reactions are at risk for anaphylaxis.

How Do I Know If My Child Is Allergic?

These allergies can't, unfortunately, be predicted by skin testing before a sting or bite occurs. The good news is that, with your help, insect allergies can be diagnosed.

The most important tool for diagnosing an insect allergy is the tale of the reaction itself. When your child is stung, here are three main things you need to do:

1. Remain calm. The allergist will make a diagnosis based on the information you provide, so stay focused.

2. Play detective. Help the doctor recreate the scene of the sting. What was your child doing where and when the sting took place? What time of day was he stung? If the insect can't be kept, then note the insect's color, presence or absence of fur, or whether the stinger was left behind.

3. Inform the doctor. Tell your child's allergist everything you can remember about your child's physical response. How did he react and how quickly did it happen? Catalogue all of the symptoms and be sure to tell the doctor if your child was on any medication at the time of the bite. If any treatment was given, tell the allergist what was administered and how your child responded to it.

Ouch!

◆ ◆ ◆ ◆ ◆

The most common insect stings come from wasps, yellow jackets, hornets and honeybees, although stings from the fire ant are becoming more frequent.

Further Diagnosis

Your child's doctor may be able to make a diagnosis based on the details of your account alone. If not, there are other diagnostic tools — primarily a skin or blood test.

Skin test. Once your child has been stung or bitten by an insect, a skin test can be highly effective. If the story of the sting sounds like something that doctors refer to as a generalized reaction — one that involves body parts away from the actual site of the sting — this skin prick test will help identify the involved insect and if other insects could potentially cause an allergic reaction. If the response, no matter how large, is localized, evidence suggests your child is not allergic and doctors will advise against skin testing, which may give false positive results.

Blood test. When skin testing isn't possible, then blood tests like the RAST may also be helpful. Once the diagnosis of an insect allergy is made, recommendations for treatment and prevention of future stings are made.

Swat It

◆ ◆ ◆ ◆ ◆

A skin test may pinpoint what insect may have caused your child's allergic reaction.

A Real Stinger

If a child has had a severe generalized reaction to a sting or bite, the risk of having an allergic reaction as bad or even worse with the next sting is 60 to 70 percent. (Children who develop only generalized hives following a sting have only a 10 percent chance of an anaphylactic reaction with subsequent stings.)

The Hit List: Most Common Insect Allergies

The stinging insects that cause the most serious allergic reactions come from the *hymenoptera*, which can be divided into two families — aphids and vespids. Here's what you need to look for:

Aphids have hairy bodies with yellow and black markings. The bumblebee is a rare offender. The honeybee leaves its stinger embedded in the skin and dies.

Yellow jackets have the yellow and black markings of a bee, but the elongated body of a small hornet. They nest in small holes in the ground or under logs. They can be quite aggressive and are the most common cause of stings in most regions of the United States and Canada.

The yellow hornet and white-faced hornet are grey and oval, looking much like their brother the yellow jacket, but bigger and with dark bands under their eyes. They nest in trees and under the eaves of houses.

Wasps have a hairless body with a narrow waist and black or brown markings. Look for them in trees and in and under eaves troughs. In colder weather, they'll take refuge in attics and closets and can be quite aggressive when they are discovered.

The fire ant (found in the southern United States) can cause anaphylaxis.

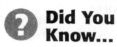 **Did You Know...**

There have been rare reports of anaphylaxis reactions from deerflies, kissing bugs, bed bugs and mosquitoes.

Treating Insect Bites and Stings

6 STEPS FOR TREATING LOCAL (NONALLERGIC) REACTIONS

1. Clean the site of the sting with a mild soap and water.

2. Apply a cool compress to the site of swelling in the first few hours after the bite.

3. Reduce the risk of infection by minimizing the amount of rubbing and scratching.

4. Relieve the itch with oral antihistamines or a corticosteroid cream or ointment.

5. Painkillers may be needed occasionally.

6. For large local reactions that are persistent, oral corticosteroids (for example, Prednisone) may be required.

GENERALIZED (ALLERGIC) REACTIONS

The treatment for a generalized reaction is an epinephrine injection. Epinephrine is another name for adrenaline, which is naturally produced by the body during stressful situations. The pre-loaded injection can be given by nonmedically trained people or by your child himself, if he's properly trained and comfortable using it. (See *Chapter 10: Coping With Allergies*, "Using The EpiPen: 5 Steps" for more information.) The EpiPen is a pre-loaded epinephrine injector prescribed by your child's doctor.

The most important treatment during a serious allergic reaction is early administration of epinephrine. You should inject epinephrine if you see any of the following signs:

Stinging Families

◆ ◆ ◆ ◆ ◆

Aphids
- Honeybee
- Bumblebee

Vespids
- Yellow jacket
- Yellow hornet
- White-faced hornet
- Wasp

- Rapidly spreading hives over the body

- Swelling in any area of the body away from the site of the sting

- Coughing, gagging, vomiting

- Throat tightness, difficulty breathing

- Dizziness, feeling faint, loss of consciousness

Note: After giving epinephrine, your child must be taken immediately to a hospital for a medical assessment; his symptoms may recur regardless of the initial treatment. In rare circumstances, your child may require a second injection within 10 to 20 minutes after the first one, but only if she is not improving or getting worse. (Children who are more than 20 minutes away from an emergency room should carry an extra epinephrine injector.) Other treatments, such as oxygen and intravenous medications, may be administered in the hospital, and your child's vital signs (heart rate, breathing rate, level of consciousness, etc.) will have to be regularly monitored.

Practice Prevention

It's happened once and that was bad enough. So how do you prevent an anaphylactic reaction from happening again? Once an insect allergy has been diagnosed, there are two ways to prevent further serious episodes:

1. Avoid further stings.

2. Reduce the severity of a reaction with allergy needles.

Timing Is Everything!

◆ ◆ ◆ ◆ ◆

If your child is allergic, the early administration of an EpiPen (epinephrine) could save his life. Get your child into the habit of wearing her EpiPen on her body at all times.

1. AVOIDANCE IS THE BEST MEDICINE.

The best way to protect your child from anaphylactic reactions is to stop the sting from ever happening. Here's how:

✓ Keep him away from any areas known to have infestations. Have any known or suspected nests around the home exterminated by trained professionals. During the spring and summer months, routinely check the house and garden for nests. Be cautious around bushes, eaves and attics.

✓ In public areas, keep your child well away from trash containers. At home, keep garbage well wrapped and covered.

✓ Shake out towels and clothing that have been left on the ground — insects may be in the folds.

✓ Do not allow your child to drink directly from a soft drink or juice can that has been sitting outside because insects may be inside.

✓ Before putting your child into a car, check for insects and always drive with windows closed.

✓ Avoid orchards and fields, particularly when they are in bloom.

✓ Discourage your child from kicking at rotting logs or bushes.

✓ Dress her in long-sleeved shirts, long pants, socks and shoes when in grass or fields.

✓ Choose white or light-colored clothes. Black and dark colors attract insects.

✓ Avoid cosmetics, perfumes and hair sprays.

✓ Keep insecticides readily available — at home and in the car — so that stinging insects can be killed from a distance.

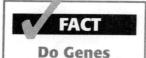

FACT

Do Genes Matter?

Allergic children, especially those with asthma, may have more severe reactions to a sting. However, a family history of insect allergies does not necessarily put your child at increased risk.

✓ If an insect lands on your child, coax him to stay still while you gently brush it away. Have him practice doing the same.

2. ALLERGY SHOTS

Immunotherapy, or allergy shots, are controversial in the treatment of some allergies, but are recommended for the prevention of severe allergic reactions to insect stings. Immunotherapy involves multiple shots with increasing amounts of insect venom to desensitize the patient to the venom. It is time consuming and expensive and, therefore, only used for children considered high risk — those who have had one serious reaction and who consequently have a 60 to 70 percent chance of a life-threatening reaction if stung again. Here's how they work:

- Starting with very low doses, venom extract is injected weekly in gradually increasing amounts.

- Once the patient is receiving an amount of venom equal to that in one to two insect stings, the frequency of injections is cut back gradually to once every eight or 12 weeks.

- This form of therapy provides up to 95 percent protection, but it must be continued for three to five years, or until the patient no longer reacts positively to skin or blood tests.

- If the patient had lost consciousness, experienced a drop in blood pressure and/or swelling in the upper airway passages with the first attack and the skin test is still positive, allergy shots are given indefinitely.

- Children who have been rendered unconscious by an insect sting should receive quarterly allergy shots for life.

Shots Alternative

◆ ◆ ◆ ◆ ◆

Allergy shots aren't for everyone. Only children who have had a life-threatening reaction and positive venom skin tests should receive shots. Children with large local reactions or generalized hives do not require shots — their subsequent reactions are usually the same or less severe.

Chapter

8

DRUG ALLERGIES

Adverse Reactions to Medications

ADVERSE REACTIONS TO DRUGS ARE MORE common than you might think, occurring almost 15 out of every 100 times that drugs are prescribed by a doctor. The World Health Organization defines an adverse reaction to a drug as "any noxious, unintended, and undesired effect of a drug that occurs at doses used for prevention, diagnosis, or treatment." However, not every adverse reaction is an allergic reaction. In fact, a true allergic response will occur in only six to 10 percent of cases in which undesirable symptoms are seen.

WHAT IS A DRUG ALLERGY?

A drug allergy is an unpredictable, unexpected adverse reaction to a drug involving IgE antibodies.

 Did You Know...

Your child's reaction to a drug can be immediate (within one hour), accelerated (1 to 72 hours) or late (days to weeks).

Nonallergic Adverse Reactions

Before deciding that your child is allergic to a drug, his doctor will want to rule out the myriad other possibilities. Children can respond negatively to a drug for a variety of reasons, including:

Toxicity. When too much of the drug is taken/used.

Side effects. These are often unavoidable, and are usually well described by the manufacturer on the drug packaging, even when using the medication according to the instructions. For example, stomach cramps are usually associated with taking some antibiotics.

Intolerance. Certain individuals may experience more severe side effects than typical side effects experienced by others. They will be forced to find an alternative medication.

Drug interactions. When two or more different drugs are taken together, one may interfere with the action of the other. (It's critical that parents inform doctors and pharmacists of other medications — both prescription and non-prescription, such as vitamins, herbal remedies, ASAs, antihistamines and laxatives.)

Allergies. A specific type of adverse reaction occurring in an extremely small number of cases. These reactions will be the main focus of this chapter.

Why *My* Child?

At the present time, there's no way of knowing which child will develop this immune response to a drug and which one won't. Allergic reactions to drugs can occur on the first exposure or when a child has had previous exposure to a drug or related substance, whether the exposure was short- or long-term. That historical experience with a medication stimulates the development of a specific immune response that doctors call an allergic response. These reactions are unpredictable and can be just as serious for children as for adults. If your child has allergic problems, such as hay fever, asthma or eczema, he isn't more likely to have a drug allergy than anyone else. However, if he has any of these disorders, his drug reaction can be more severe. The reasons for such reactions are not completely understood.

Action Reaction

◆ ◆ ◆ ◆ ◆

Allergic reactions to a drug are unpredictable and occur in a small number of patients.

How Do I Know If My Child Is Allergic?

There are several different forms of immune responses, but the most common involves the production of a specific antibody called Immunoglobulin E (IgE). This type of reaction is called the Type-1 allergic reaction. When that antibody is present, you may have one or more of the following symptoms:

- Rashes, including hives

- Swelling of the deeper tissues (angioedema)

- Anaphylaxis, a rare and more severe form of an allergic reaction. In addition to the symptoms above, anaphylaxis includes difficulty breathing and a drop in blood pressure

Antibiotics

Of all the drug allergies, allergic response to antibiotics is by far the most common among allergic individuals. And it's within that family of drugs, penicillin, or a related drug, amoxicillin, that there seems to be the most prevalent problems. That makes good sense when you consider that penicillin is the most widely prescribed antibiotic in the world. However, 80 percent of patients who think they have an allergy to penicillin actually have reactions for other reasons, such as rashes from the infection that the antibiotic had initially been prescribed for.

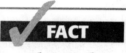

FACT

The Real Culprit?

As many as 17 percent of patients tell their doctors they are allergic to penicillin, while only 1 to 2 percent have a true allergy. And of these, only a very small number will have a very serious reaction, or anaphylaxis.

TESTING FOR PENICILLIN ALLERGIES

Fortunately, there is very reliable testing available to diagnose a penicillin allergy. An allergist will conduct skin prick tests on your child's forearm. If these tests are negative, then the allergist will inject a small amount of penicillin just under the skin on your child's arm. If the skin test shows a positive result, the testing is stopped and the patient is diagnosed as having a penicillin allergy. But if the skin test is negative, an oral dose of penicillin is often given. This 'oral challenge' is a very reliable way of completing the assessment for a penicillin allergy. (See *Chapter 1: Introduction to Allergies* for an explanation of these tests.)

3 ACTIONS YOU SHOULD TAKE WHEN YOUR CHILD IS ALLERGIC

1. Inform your child's doctor.

2. Inform all of your child's caregivers, including medical caregivers.

3. Have your child wear a MedicAlert bracelet or necklace clearly stating his allergy to penicillin and medications in that family.

MEET THE PENICILLIN FAMILY

If your child is allergic to penicillin, he should not be given any of the drugs in the penicillin family. This includes:

- Penicillin
- Amoxicillin
- Ampicillin
- Piperacillin
- Pondocillin
- Cloxacillin

There are a few others in the family that are less commonly used and should also be avoided.

Penicillin Tolerance

◆ ◆ ◆ ◆ ◆

About 97 to 99 percent of children who complete the oral challenge with a negative response will tolerate penicillin with no risk of a Type-1 allergic response.

DESENSITIZATION TO PENICILLIN

There are rare cases in which children are infected with life-threatening diseases for which penicillin is the *only* drug of choice. Should this happen, and your child is allergic to penicillin, doctors may suggest a procedure called 'desensitization,' which will allow your child to tolerate a full course of treatment for that particular infection only.

What Is Desensitization?

An extremely small amount of the suspecting drug is administered, with increasing doses given very slowly every 20 minutes until the patient can tolerate the full dose. The whole process takes only a few hours; in rare circumstances, it may be done over a period of several days.

The desensitization procedure must be done in a hospital and is only good for the current course of antibiotics — it would have to be repeated, should your child require penicillin in the future.

Related Sensitivities: The Cephalosporins

If your child is allergic to penicillin, he may have an allergic reaction to a family of antibiotics called cephalosporins. This family shares a similar structure called the ß-lactam ring with the penicillin family, putting allergic children at risk for cross-reactivity. The exact percentage of cross-reactions is unknown, but is thought to be quite low.

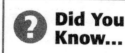
Unfortunately, there is no reliable skin testing available for cephalosporin allergy. The best you can do is avoid this family of medications and have your child wear a MedicAlert bracelet.

If a situation arises in which the only medication suitable for a particular infection is one of the cephalosporins, your doctor may want to administer a procedure called **provocative testing**.

Provocative testing involves giving incremental doses of the desired antibiotic over a short period of time and under close observation. Your doctor is actually trying to 'provoke' an allergic response. Should none exist, he may safely prescribe a cephalosporin drug. But if your child does develop an allergic response, your doctor may choose to proceed with desensitization (see the box on the opposite page).

ALL IN THE FAMILY

Children suspected of having a cephalosporin allergy should have complete penicillin testing done to ensure that they are not also allergic to the penicillin family of medications.

MEET THE CEPHALOSPORIN FAMILY

The cephalosporin family of antibiotics includes:

- Cefprozil (Cefzil)
- Cefuroxime (Ceftin)
- Cefaclor (Ceclor)
- Cephalexin (Keflex)

Nonsteroidal Anti-inflammatory Drugs (NSAIDs)

You and I call them Aspirin and Motrin and we use them for everything from mild pain relief to fever reduction. But doctors call these over-the-counter drugs nonsteroidal anti-inflammatory drugs (NSAIDs). Included in this class of medications are acetylsalicylic acid (Aspirin), ibuprofen (Motrin) and naproxen (Naprosyn).

Reactions to NSAIDs do occur and, in rare situations, can also cause anaphylaxis. If your child is diagnosed with an allergy to a specific NSAID, it must be avoided. (And as with other medication allergies, your child should wear a MedicAlert bracelet or necklace at all times.) But fortunately, with so many options available in this class of drugs, safe alternatives can usually be found for your child. In the few instances when a child demonstrates an allergy to all members of the NSAID family, a desensitization process may be required.

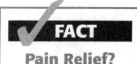

FACT

Pain Relief?

There are many adverse reactions to NSAIDs that are not allergic. Some children with asthma, for example, can experience a worsening of their symptoms after ingesting Aspirin. Others who suffer chronic hives may find that their hives worsen when they ingest an NSAID.

Anaesthetics

LOCAL ANAESTHETICS

This group of medications is used to decrease the pain involved during dental procedures and other minor procedures, such as stitching a cut. Commonly used local anaesthetics include: lidocaine (xylocaine), tetracaine, bupivacaine and many others. These medications are injected locally into the skin. Adverse reactions to local anaesthetics occur less than one percent of the time. But when they do occur, the majority of reactions are nonallergic and are mainly caused by:

1. *Manipulation of the tissues,* causing localized swelling.

2. *Reactions to an additive* called epinephrine, contained in some local anaesthetics. It causes increased heart rate, increased blood pressure and irregular heart rate.

3. *Psychological reactions* in which children have some symptoms of panic that can mimic an allergic reaction.

TESTING FOR LOCAL ANAESTHETICS ALLERGIES

If your child has any type of reaction to a local anaesthetic, testing by a certified allergist may be in order to rule out future problems. Typically, an allergist will start with a **skin prick test**, then proceed to **intradermal** testing — in which a small amount of dilute anaesthetic is injected just under the skin. (See *Chapter 1: Introduction to Allergies* for more information on these tests.) If the child shows no adverse reactions, the doctor will continue by administering a full dose of the anaesthetic.

If all tests are negative, a letter can be sent to your child's doctor clearly specifying the anaesthetic your child is safe to use.

Testing isn't necessary if the anaesthetic that caused the initial reaction is known. Because there are two major groups of anaesthetic medications, often a safe alternative can be chosen without any further testing since the two groups of medication are quite different and don't cross-react.

Be An Informant

◆ ◆ ◆ ◆ ◆

Before visiting any doctor's office, bring the name of the exact medication or a copy of the treatment record of the drug that caused your child's reaction.

GENERAL ANAESTHETICS

If your child has experienced allergy-like symptoms during a surgical procedure, it's likely a response to one of the many other substances administered or involved in a surgical process. (See "General Alert.")

The safest course of action is to have your child evaluated by an allergist. Skin testing can be done to determine which of the many medications used by the anesthetist is the cause of adverse symptoms. It's essential to avoid any medications with positive results to ensure safety of future general anesthesia.

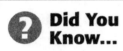 **Did You Know...**

Allergic reactions from a general anaesthetic occur between 1 in 5,000 and 1 in 15,000 cases.

General Alert

Anesthetists use a variety of medications in any single surgery and any one of them could be the culprit in an allergic reaction. One of the more common ones is called muscle relaxants. Before you blame the anesthetic itself, the doctor has to also rule out other substances, which are also used in surgical procedures. They include:

- Pain killers
- Hypnotics
- Latex
- Sedatives
- Antibiotics

VACCINES

Vaccinations, or immunizations, are one of the most important preventive medical advancements of our time, literally wiping out some infectious diseases, like smallpox, while protecting us against the suffering that goes along with other illnesses. In North America, there are very specific guidelines around immunizations for children; the goal is to not only protect each individual child but to also protect the 'herd' (all children). There is extremely good evidence that the very existence of certain infectious diseases has declined dramatically since immunizing began, as have associated complications, including death. That's why immunizations are so strongly advised — and are even mandatory for children in some areas.

But what if your child is allergic to the immunization meant to protect her? While such allergies are extremely uncommon, they do happen. The allergist can take a detailed history of the reaction to a vaccine, and, if necessary, perform a skin prick test and intradermal testing similar to the one done with drug allergies described on page 153. Then, the doctor may offer a decision based on the results of the skin testing. A desensitization procedure might be used in some cases in order to safely administer the vaccine.

VACCINATIONS WITH EGG SOURCES

In the not-too-distant past, parents of children with egg allergy were cautioned against the MMR (measles, mumps, rubella) vaccine, along with the vaccine for influenza. That's because these vaccines are derived from egg sources. But the Canadian Immunization Guidelines state clearly that patients with egg allergy *can* now safely receive the MMR vaccine without any special testing, because the amount of egg protein is extremely small and therefore inconsequential. However, you should consult your child's physician before he receives the influenza immunization, since it contains a larger amount of egg protein, which varies from year to year.

> ## Covering All Cracks
>
> ◆ ◆ ◆ ◆ ◆
>
> Today, fewer and fewer vaccines are prepared with egg proteins, However, it's important to ask the doctor about any egg protein additive before your child receives a particular vaccination.

Chapter

9

LATEX ALLERGY

Allergy to Natural Rubber

SINCE THE EARLY 1980S, THE USE OF LATEX in the health-care profession has increased significantly. At the time, latex gloves were seen as a superior product to other gloves being produced at the time because of their strength, elasticity and tactile sensitivity, as well as their effectiveness against the spread of infection and the AIDS virus. Unfortunately, as the demand for latex gloves soared, so did the reports of abnormal reactions to latex, which ranged from mild skin rashes to life-threatening anaphylaxis. The exact reasons for the rise of this allergy are not completely understood.

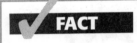

✔ FACT

A Leading Role

Over the past 20 years, natural rubber latex has become a significant allergy problem. The rise coincides with the growing use of latex over the last two decades.

WHAT IS A LATEX ALLERGY?

Children who are allergic to latex can have a reaction when they touch or breath in latex, or come in contact with an individual who regularly uses latex gloves or products. An allergy to latex causes similar reactions as other allergies. Symptoms can include:

- Itching

- Swelling

- Rash or hives

- Sneezing

- Congested or runny nose

- Difficulty breathing (in more severe cases)

What Is Latex?

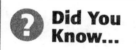
Natural rubber latex, also referred to as latex, is commonly used to make medical supplies, household products and toys. It comes from the sap of the rubber tree (*Hevea brasiliensis*) found primarily in Africa and Southeast Asia. Chemicals are added to its sap, heated and treated to produce elastic products. Porcelain molds are dipped into the treated sap to also produce various thin products such as balloons and gloves. (See "Not All Rubber is Equal" for a list of items that may contain latex.)

Not All Rubber Is Equal

Unlike natural rubber, synthetic rubber is made from butyl or petroleum components, and does not contain latex. Therefore, material made of synthetic rubber doesn't pose the same allergic threat as natural rubber. Stretchable or elastic products, such as gloves or balloons, are a major source of problems. Latex is also often used to make:

- Baby bottle nipples, pacifiers
- Toys, such as balloons, balls, playground equipment
- Bicycle handle grips; taped tennis racquet handles
- Bandages
- Hot water bottles
- Erasers
- Sports gear
- Rubber bands
- Condoms
- Medical products such as Band-Aids, first-aid tape, syringes, tubing and catheters

Latex Contact

Reactions to latex can occur in many different settings, in particular, medical procedures such as vaginal examinations and barium enemas, dental procedures, X-rays and during abdominal, urinary or genital surgery.

In hospitals, parents may be concerned about the possible allergy risk of rubber in certain medical equipment, such as injection ports, rubber stoppers, gas masks and blood pressure cuffs. However, because of even small amounts of latex in products and their potential for release after repeated washings, hospitals have opted to use non-latex alternatives. Today, most of these items either contain very small amounts of latex or other types of rubber that don't have the same allergic risk.

Breathing In

◆ ◆ ◆ ◆ ◆

In some environments, latex may be inhaled. Powder on latex gloves, for example, can carry the latex protein particles — which cause the allergy reaction — through inhaling.

Symptoms of Latex Allergy

If your child comes in contact with latex, he may experience a number of symptoms, depending on the body's response.

CONTACT REACTIONS
Irritant Contact Dermatitis

The typical signs of irritant contact dermatitis include hand redness, dryness, cracking, scaling and blisters. While these reactions are not caused by an allergic reaction to latex, they can occur from sweating and rubbing the area that makes contact under the glove, from repeated washing and drying, and from residual soaps and detergents that remain on the skin for a long period of time.

Allergic Contact Dermatitis

This is a specific immune response with eczema-like rashes and blisters on the backs of the hands. The lesions typically appear 48 to 96 hours after exposure. The skin may become dry, crusted and thickened with continued exposure to latex. Many of the chemical products added during the glove manufacturing process, such as thiuram, thiazole, carbamate, are to blame.

When latex is rubbed off from the gloves by sweat or other body fluids, latex can be transferred from nicks in the skin's surface into the body. In this instance, latex proteins, and not the chemical additives, are what is transferred through the skin. This transfer can increase the risk of latex sensitization, cause subsequent reactions in other areas of the body and even produce life-threatening reactions.

✔ **FACT**

High Alert

Up to 30 percent of latex-sensitive children can have a life-threatening allergic reaction.

REACTIONS IN OTHER BODY AREAS

When latex proteins are transferred to other parts of the body, skin reactions, such as hives with or without swelling of the skin, are common. Other reactions that involve internal surfaces or openings, such as the eyes, nose and mouth, can manifest as a congested runny nose or red watery eyes, asthma, anaphylaxis and even death.

High-risk Groups

Children with spina bifida or chronic urologic abnormalities. This group is frequently exposed to natural rubber because of various procedures used to manage their condition, such as X-rays and surgeries. It's recommended that children with such conditions avoid exposure to latex products early in life.

Children who have undergone multiple surgical procedures. In particular, children requiring frequent surgical or complex reconstructive procedures for birth defects may be at risk of developing a latex allergy.

A history of anaphylaxis of unknown or uncertain cause. Allergic reactions of unknown cause should be thoroughly evaluated, and latex allergy suspected in any patient who has had a previous unexplained anaphylactic reaction during a surgical, dental or investigative procedure, such as X-rays.

History of other allergies (food allergies, asthma, allergic rhinitis, eczema). Allergic patients are more likely to develop a latex allergy. The type and severity of an allergy does not correlate directly with the nature and degree of latex hypersensitivity. However, there are certain relationships:

- Many individuals allergic to latex are also sensitive to fruits (banana, kiwi, avocado) and nuts (chestnuts). The reverse (those with fruit sensitivities being allergic to latex) is less common.

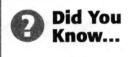 **Did You Know...**

Research shows that from 67 percent to 73 percent of children with spina bifida or severe abnormalities in the urinary or genital areas have an allergy to latex.

- Individuals with eczema or dermatitis, especially involving the hands, who are exposed to latex gloves are also at high risk for sensitization because the latex proteins can be transferred through the cracks in their hands.

- Asthma sufferers aren't predisposed to anaphylaxis, but their symptoms can become severe if exposed to latex and if they are sensitive to latex. Asthmatic symptoms, which include coughing, congestion and chest tightness as well as wheezing, need to be controlled in latex-sensitive individuals.

Health-care workers. Medical/dental personnel and other health-care workers (about five to 17 percent) who are routinely exposed to natural rubber latex in their working environments are at higher risk.

Occupational exposure to latex. Individuals working in fields with exposure to rubber, a surgical glove manufacturing plant, greenhouses, latex doll manufacturing plant and a textile factory, are all constantly exposed to latex and at risk of developing an allergy to it.

Female gender. The exact reasons why women are more prone to a latex allergy over men is not clear but it may be related to more extensive occupational exposure, especially in the health-care field, and a greater degree of mucosal contact with latex antigen from contraceptives and routine obstetric/gynecological procedures.

Take-out Tip

◆ ◆ ◆ ◆ ◆

When eating out, ask your server or the kitchen if latex gloves are used to prepare certain foods.

Allergy Testing

WHO SHOULD BE TESTED?

Your child could be a candidate for further testing if he experiences any one of these symptoms or fits into any of the categories outlined in the section "High-risk Groups" on the previous pages. Of course, if your child is about to undergo any medical, surgical, X-ray or dental procedure where gloves might be used, ensure the doctor/technician has asked you questions to determine whether your child fits into any of these high-risk groups.

TESTING: MAKING A DIAGNOSIS

Skin tests. In the skin prick test, the superficial skin layers are pricked and a drop of extract is added (see *Chapter 1: Introduction to Allergies,* page 34 for more information on the testing procedure). Sometimes various glove preparations instead of the commercial extract are applied directly on the skin, particularly when the history is very convincing and the skin test is negative. If these tests still show a negative result, then a clinician might recommend wearing a latex glove for 15 to 20 minutes and observing if a rash develops on the hand.

Blood tests. Specific testing like the latex radioallergosorbent test (RAST) can be quite helpful for specific populations such as those with spina bifida, especially if they have experienced anaphylaxis. Other blood tests, such as the ImmunoCap and the AlaSTAT, can be helpful when the skin test is negative, but they also can't identify the allergy 100 percent of the time.

 Did You Know...

Many products that used to be made of latex are now being made with other materials, such as neoprene. But if you're not sure about the material in a product, call its manufacturer and ask if it's safe for your child.

Note: All of these tests are very helpful when the reactions are severe, but results are less helpful when symptoms are less dramatic. If your child has less specific symptoms, especially if he's in a high-risk category, speak to the child's physician about the history of her reactions before determining what type of tests to undergo.

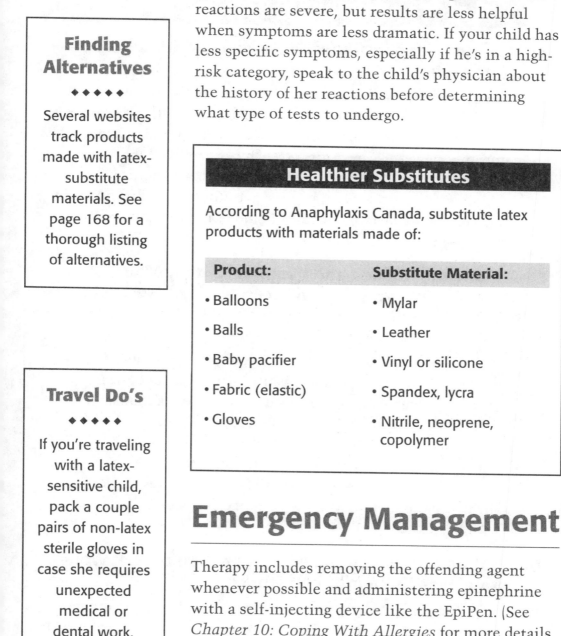

Finding Alternatives

◆ ◆ ◆ ◆ ◆

Several websites track products made with latex-substitute materials. See page 168 for a thorough listing of alternatives.

Travel Do's

◆ ◆ ◆ ◆ ◆

If you're traveling with a latex-sensitive child, pack a couple pairs of non-latex sterile gloves in case she requires unexpected medical or dental work.

Healthier Substitutes

According to Anaphylaxis Canada, substitute latex products with materials made of:

Product:	Substitute Material:
• Balloons	• Mylar
• Balls	• Leather
• Baby pacifier	• Vinyl or silicone
• Fabric (elastic)	• Spandex, lycra
• Gloves	• Nitrile, neoprene, copolymer

Emergency Management

Therapy includes removing the offending agent whenever possible and administering epinephrine with a self-injecting device like the EpiPen. (See *Chapter 10: Coping With Allergies* for more details on how to administer this device.) Children allergic to latex should always carry the EpiPen device.

LATEX-SAFE ENVIRONMENTS — Q & A

Q: How do I keep my latex-sensitive child from getting a latex reaction?

A: The only certain measure that can avert a serious allergic reaction to latex rubber is avoiding latex products altogether. But that's not always easy — thousands of products are made with latex, not all companies have the capability to replace or remove rubber from their products, and product labeling is often inadequate or incomplete. Parents with latex-sensitive children are encouraged to also eliminate latex products at home or in other environments when possible.

Q: Are doctors' offices and hospitals a dangerous place for my five-year-old recently diagnosed with a latex allergy?

A: Most health-care facilities and hospitals, which in the past had high exposure to latex, have recently adopted a hospital-safe environment. The designation ensures that products containing latex are eliminated and/or replaced with non-latex items. Of course, these hospitals are also prepared to recognize and treat any allergic reaction from a hidden source of latex. If your child has a doctor's appointment, notify the health-care professionals of his allergy and ask the office to schedule you as the first patient of the day to minimize exposure to airborne powdered latex gloves.

Q: What advice do you have for people who must work with gloves in their line of work?

A: People who are required to wear gloves and are in direct contact with latex-allergic individuals should only wear non-latex gloves. If you work with a latex-sensitive individual, it is safe for you to wear gloves that have a low level of latex and no powder.

Q: How can I ensure people around my child are aware of her allergy to latex?

A: Make sure your child carries some form of identification, such as a MedicAlert bracelet, that indicates she is latex-sensitive. If your child is hospitalized, ask the facility to post warning signs of her allergy on the rooms where she's being treated.

Q. Where can I get more information about products that have latex in them?

A: Various dedicated Internet sites provide information about latex allergies, as well as lists of latex and non-latex items to help individuals keep track of potentially hazardous products. (See our chart following this page and our Resources section, starting on page 238, for several sites). For example, many latex-based paints are no longer a concern. If you're still not sure about whether a product contains latex, call the company that makes the item and enquire about its latex content.

Latex-Free Gloves?

Just because some gloves are labeled "hypoallergenic" don't assume they're a suitable alternative to latex gloves. Measurable latex allergen levels have been found in these gloves. The hypoallergenic label, in this instance, refers to a reduction in the additive chemicals responsible for contact dermatitis, and NOT a reduction in latex-sensitive proteins.

LATEX ALTERNATIVES

Many products may contain latex. Make your child's environment latex-free with these possible alternatives.

May Contain Latex	Examples of Latex-free Alternatives
Automobile (floor mats, steering wheel)	Vinyl; clear; leather
Art supplies (paint, markers, glue)	See www.latexallergyresources.org/ Product_lists/school_products.cfm
Balloons	Mylar balloons
Balls (koosh, tennis, rubber, basketball)	Vinyl; Thorton sports balls; PVC-Hedstrom sports ball
Bandages	Curad; Kendall; SciVolutions; Phoenix Health Care Products
Bath mat	Bathroom throw rugs with non-skid latex backing); 100% cotton reversible rug (Lands End)
Braces or splints with foam lining	Line with cloth or felt
Chewing gum	Bubblicious, Trident, Dentyne, Mint A Burst, Cinn A Burst, Fruit A Burst (Warner-Lambert); Wrigley's Gums
Cold wraps & latex-free packaging	Phoenix Health Care Products
Condoms, diaphragms, contraceptive sponge	Durex Avanti; Trojan Supra; Reality female condom; Silicone Diaphragm (Milex)
Cosmetics, applicators, sponges, eye lash curler, waterproof mascara	Use cotton balls or brushes; All Natural Cosmetics (Cosmetics Without Synthetics); Clinique; Luminescence

Note: Cosmetics may contain papain, a papaya derivative that can cross react with latex

Crutches (axillary & hand pads)	Cover with Stockinette, cloth or tape)

May Contain Latex	Examples of Latex-free Alternatives
Disposable diapers,	Huggies, Pull-Ups, Goodnites
Earphones, headsets	Earplugs (Lyons Safety)
Elastic, underwear, clothing	Cover with cloth; products by Decent Exposures; Elan Patterns & Supplies; BlueCanoe; Seventh Generation
Feeding nipples	Silicone Gerber; Evenflo; MAM; Mead Johnson; some products by Russ
Feminine sanitary pads and tampons	New Freedom (Kimberly-Clark); TAMPAX Naturals; NatraCare
Floor coverings, carpet backing, mats	Wooden floors; provide barrier cloth; The Stopper; Non-skid rug pad
Foam rubber	Synthetic foam
Food storage bags/ zippered plastic bags	Wax paper; plain plastic bags; Ziploc Dow Brands; HandiWrap; Saran Wrap
Garden hoses	Use vinyl ones
Gloves (housekeeping, rubber, kitchen)	Heavy duty nitrile (Lyons Safety); Vinyl Allerderm; Nyplex (Magla); Solvex nitryl (Ansell); products by Lab Safety Supply
Gloves used with food handling	Synthetic, vinyl (inquire at grocery stores & restaurants before eating)
Glue, envelopes, stamps	Use wet cloth to moisten
Helmets, bike	Bell Sports
Insulin injections	AdvantaJet
Medical products	See http://www.latexallergyresources.org/ Product_lists/hospital_products.cfm
Mouse pad	MediaMate; FastTrac Mouse Pad Model #15640; Expressions #6292 (Rubbermaid); Keytronics; Mouse on keyboard Model # (1P)LT Trackball; Reason Technology; Levengers AD258

May Contain Latex	Examples of Latex-free Alternatives
Pacifiers	Plastic, silicone and vinyl; Infa; Gerber; MAM; Binky
Pantyhose	Tuck clothes under waist band; Lycra-Spandex; L'EGGS
Pens with rubber grips	Use plastic, carry own
Raincoats, waterproof boots	Neoprene-coated nylon, PVC Gempers
Rubber bands	Plasticbands Baumgarten
Rubber button pads on phones, calculator, TV remote	Most are silicone rubber. Check with manufacturer
School supplies	See www.latexallergyresources.org/ Product_lists/school_products.cfm
Shoes (rubber boots, crepe sole, archpads, thongs, water shoes)	Rubber free sport shoe (PW Minor Shoe Company); PVC waterproof boots (Gemnlers); insoles Frelonic; Superfeet
Socks	Cotton socks without elastic; Vermont Country Stor; Buster Brown; Dr. Leonards Health Care Catalogue; Kathy Ireland cotton/lycra/nylon
Spatulas	Wooden, plastic, synthetic, Pampered Chef
Sports equipment	
• Water toys	PVC or plastic
• Swim cap, thongs, goggles	Silicone swim caps; silicone or vinyl
• Wet suits, scuba/ snorkel masks & equip't	LaCosta
• Handles (ping pong paddles, Golf clubs, Aluminum baseball bat, Tennis/squash/rackets, Ski poles)	Rawling Sporting Goods; Spalding Sporting Goods; Wilson Sporting Goods

May Contain Latex	Examples of Latex-free Alternatives
Sports equipment (cont'd)	
• Canoe, Kayak, Rafting equipment	Planetary Gear

Note: WINN Inc. sells polyurethane replacement grips for sports equipment

Stretch fabrics (some)	Lycra-spandex, Dupont
Swimsuits	Suits Me Swimware
T-shirts with appliques	Tape (adhesive, scotch, masking)
Plastic, silk tape	Microfoam; Micropore; Durapore; Transpore; Dermaclear; Dermicel; Waterproof (J&J)
Tools with rubber handles	Vinyl; leather handles; cover with tape
Toothbrush handles with rubber grips, infant tooth massager	Oral B; Reach soft bristle, Crest

Note: Most of these handles are synthetic. Check with the manufacturer

Toys (rubber ducky, teething toys, etc.)	Plastic, cloth, vinyl; Jurassic Park Figures (Kenner); 1993 Barbie; Disney Dolls; See N Say (Mattel); toys by Little Tykes/Rubbermaid; Playschool; Little People Toys (Fisher-Price); Discovery Toys; Many toys made by The First Years, Shelcore, Safety First

Note: It is best to contact the manufacturer if you have any concerns. Many toys are latex free

Upholstery foam rubber padding	Synthetic foam
Wheel chair cushions, tires	Jay; ROHO; Cushions

Reprinted with permission by the American Latex Allergy Association.

Note: This list is a guideline for informational purposes only. For more information, contact the American Latex Allergy Association at alert@execpc.com or (888) 972-5378.

PART 3

Dealing with Allergies & Asthma

Chapter

10

COPING WITH ALLERGIES

Educating Your Children and Their Caregivers

WHEN YOUR CHILD IS FIRST DIAGNOSED with allergies, it's common to experience a wide range of emotions, from confusion and frustration to anxiety, fear, guilt or even grief. Keeping these emotions in check will help you to restore a sense of balance in your life and enable you to live with your child's allergies. Here, in this chapter, we focus on tips to help you cope with your child's allergies. For additional information, see our *Resources* section at the end of this book.

Restoring the Balance

Whether your child has been diagnosed with asthma, eczema, hay fever, anaphylaxis or allergies to food, insects, dust, pollen, latex, medications or even the family pet, it's important to know that life doesn't have to stop. Your child's allergies may require extra demands on your family, but with a little extra planning and education you'll soon find life to be manageable once again.

✔ **FACT**

Wide Net

About 20 to 30 percent of the population has some allergic problem.

Knowledge is Power

Allergic disorders are very common. Thankfully, you'll find a large amount of information available from many credible sources. However, some other sources may provide misinformation and foster misconceptions. Parents and patients need to know how to acquire the 'right' information for their specific medical condition. Your family doctor, pediatrician or nursing staff can assist you.

Take Charge

◆ ◆ ◆ ◆ ◆

With a wealth of resources available to you and your child, you can be in charge of his allergy problem.

In some cases, your child will need to be referred to an allergist, where you can obtain further information. Outside of the medical profession, there are several lay and professional organizations that deal with allergy problems. Most of them have informative Internet sites and offer brochures and updates on new advances. Some of these groups also hold meetings and support groups where you can share ideas and concerns with other people. Others organize various conferences where you can get a chance to meet experts in the field and ask questions.

? Did You Know...

Many organizations offer support — by joining one in your area, you can meet other parents with similar challenges and share your solutions. The national groups also have forums in their newsletters and at various conferences.

Coping with Emotions

There are a range of emotions that can overwhelm you at times. As parents, it's normal to experience some of these feelings, but it's reassuring to know that by taking control you can get back in the 'driver's seat.'

Confusion. Once you begin to gather information, you'll be bombarded with material from professional and nonprofessional sources, such as friends, family, books, magazine and newspaper articles. In many cases, much of the information is too general to apply to your specific case. There is nothing wrong with seeking as much information as possible on your child's allergic condition, provided you ask for professional advice from your doctor or a recognized organization before you start applying any concept into your child's medical treatment plan.

Frustration. Allergies often interfere and disrupt family activities, relationships and even schoolwork. At times, making special considerations for your allergic child may even cause conflicts with other siblings. Be aware of these feelings and how they're affecting your family.

Anxiety/fear. Discuss your anxieties and fears and recognize that the 'what if' questions mean that you need to get more information. For example, many children with peanut or fish allergies fear they may have a life-threatening reaction by just smelling the allergic food's fumes. This fear has been so exaggerated by public misconceptions that many allergic children are also frightened of being close to someone who is eating a peanut butter sandwich. But, a recent study found that this type of contact did not cause a reaction in peanut-sensitive children, provided they didn't ingest the food.

Guilt. It can interfere with your ability to assist your child, but it's important you don't blame yourself or feel guilty for your child's allergies. Although the tendency of developing allergies is inherited, so are your child's eye color and good looks. Remember, it's all part of the genetic package you pass along to your children and you have no control whether they develop allergies or not. So, stop blaming yourself and start taking positive action.

Grief. Both you and your child may experience it. There is often a sense of loss when allergies are diagnosed. Your child may have to carry medication, be limited to travel short distances from home and never know what it's like to cuddle up with a furry family pet. You may grieve

Lean On You

◆ ◆ ◆ ◆ ◆

Give your child the support she needs to cope with aspects of her allergic condition. For example, she may not get to eat the same things as her friends.

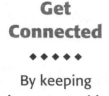

Get Connected

◆ ◆ ◆ ◆ ◆

By keeping in contact with reliable sources, you'll be able to get fast and credible verification of the 'news.'

differently, missing the simplicity of life before your child's allergies. You may have to change the way you shop for food, read food labels, clean your house, or make special arrangements for traveling. Don't blame your child or yourself for the extra demands her allergies put on your family — instead make it a point to learn more about her condition and how to balance it in everyday living.

Creative Thinking

Once you've allowed you and your child to express your feelings about living with an allergic condition, develop an action plan from credible information. In it, you'll also need to plan for unexpected situations, such as being away from home for a lengthy period. In time, you and your family will learn new and innovative ways of doing all the things you once enjoyed.

Managing Your Child's Allergies

Each child and their allergic condition vary. While one child may suffer from potentially life-threatening allergies known as anaphylaxis, another may develop an itchy rash and runny nose when petting the neighbor's cat. Whatever the case may be, developing a plan to manage your child's allergies is essential. Here are some suggestions and tips to help you get you started.

LIVING WITH ASTHMA

One of the major problems that parents and other caregivers are faced with is recognizing the more subtle signs of this condition and acting at an early stage to help the child. Failing to recognize these factors entirely can lead to serious asthmatic problems and even death.

Some parents believe that a child's condition will improve if he just 'works through an attack' by continuing to exercise and not take any medication. But this only puts the child in danger. The main goals in maintaining asthma under control are:

- Having no symptoms throughout the day or the night

- Being able to partake in normal activities with no restrictions

- Having minimal or no spontaneous flare-ups

- Not visiting the emergency department at the hospital

- Not missing school or work

- Having minimal or no medications (The use of Ventolin more than twice a week is a problem.)

- Not experiencing any side effects from medications

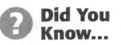 **Did You Know...**

Caregivers of asthmatic children should be aware of what helps maintain good control of their condition. Any deviation, however slight, from a child's treatment can be dangerous. (See *Chapter 2: Asthma* for more information on managing asthma.)

What Can Prompt an Episode

It's important to understand the different ways an asthmatic episode can occur, and how mild symptoms also need to be recognized and treated. Those who have other allergic problems, such as insect or peanut allergies, are at higher risk of having an episode if they encounter an allergic trigger and their asthma is not under good control.

Symptom Puzzle

◆ ◆ ◆ ◆ ◆

Not every asthmatic episode is characterized by wheezing. Some asthmatics may have repetitive or prolonged coughing, shortness of breath or chest tightness.

A Taste for Safety

◆ ◆ ◆ ◆ ◆

Don't risk a possible reaction — always avoid unlabeled foods.

LIVING WITH FOOD ALLERGIES

The challenge is to make allergens visible. In order to do this, you'll need to learn about which foods are safe or unsafe for your child, how to read a food label, and how to handle food allergy problems outside the home in certain settings, such as in restaurants, schools, camps, and when traveling.

Safe and Unsafe Foods

Safe foods include:

- **Foods prepared at home.** You can control the ingredients in dishes you make.

- **Foods labeled by a well-known North American manufacturer,** particularly one that you have contacted for information about its products.

Potentially unsafe foods include:

- **Bulk foods.** There is a high risk of cross contamination.

- **Desserts and baked goods.** Unless you are sure that they've been safely prepared, it's particularly difficult to avoid peanut, tree nut, egg and milk allergens in desserts.

- **Imported foods.** Manufacturing and labeling practices vary around the world. Most Canadian and U.S. food recalls for undeclared allergens apply to imports, mainly outside of North America.

- **Foods that are labeled "may contain."** Despite the common misconception that manufacturers place these warnings in order to protect themselves, it's not worth second-guessing whether or not a specific warning should be taken seriously.

- **Shared food, utensils, straws or containers** may contain allergens.

How To Read a Food Label

You'll also need to learn how to read a food label to ensure your child is eating safe foods. It can seem time-consuming at first, but you'll become much quicker with practice. And, you'll need to pass along your expertise to your child so she's always aware of what she's eating.

Here's what you'll need to know to understand a food label:

- **Learn alternate names for your allergen(s).** At the time of writing, North American manufacturers have not yet been required to use plain language on food labels. If you're looking for the presence of milk, for example, you'll need to know that milk protein can also be listed as *whey* or *casein*. Likewise, *ovalbumin* implies the presence of egg. (See charts, starting on page 111.)

- **Get to know the manufacturer** and stay with those companies that have a good reputation for handling allergens.

- **Read the label every time.** Manufacturing practices can change at any time and without notice.

- **Be aware of the differences in labeling practices** when traveling to other countries.

- **Sign up to receive notices of food recalls.** In Canada, this service is provided through Anaphylaxis Canada and the Canadian Food Inspection Agency. In the States, contact The Food Allergy & Anaphylaxis Network.

Visiting Restaurants

If you've avoided taking your children to a restaurant because of the potential for a reaction, take note. While allergic reactions are common in restaurants,

---

Label Language

♦ ♦ ♦ ♦ ♦

Don't forget that label warnings have their limitations. The absence of a warning doesn't imply that the food is safe.

Proceed with Caution

♦ ♦ ♦ ♦ ♦

Review **allergy-free** claims. Your definition of allergen-free and the manufacturer's definition may not mean the same thing. For example, there have been reports of reactions to trace amounts of milk in "milk-free" Pareve products and traces of tree nuts in "peanut-free" products.

they usually occur because of a patron's failure to ask the right questions or ask the right people.

If you're uncomfortable with any of the answers you receive in a restaurant, it's best to leave the locale so it sends a strong message to your child that you will not take any chances. It also helps them feel more secure.

When eating out:

✓ Call ahead of time and speak to a manager about how they handle food allergies.

✓ Dine during 'off hours' when the restaurant and staff are not as busy. Some establishments will even be able to set up for your child's birthday party during these off hours.

✓ Ask if it's possible to inspect the kitchen and speak to the chef directly.

✓ Don't expect the waiter or waitress to understand your child's allergy at the same level you do.

✓ Ask to read their food labels and speak directly to the person who will be preparing your child's food.

Making Allergens a Priority

In Canada, 10 'priority allergens' must be labeled, or the product is subject to a recall. The list includes: peanut, tree nuts, egg, milk, soy, wheat, fish, crustaceans, sesame and sulfites greater than 10 parts per million. If the allergen you're concerned about isn't one of the 10, you can't assume that absence from the label implies absence from the product. For more information, Anaphylaxis Canada or The Food Allergy & Anaphylaxis Network in the United States have created a series of allergen information cards that can help you navigate labels safely.

LIVING WITH ANAPHYLAXIS

A diagnosis of a serious allergy is a life-changing event. Unlike a passing illness, an allergy may never go away and can disrupt your family's life in many ways. It demands your full attention and full response. The effects of denial can be disastrous, especially in the case of anaphylaxis.

As difficult as things may seem at first, it's possible to live safely and fully with potentially life-threatening allergies. In order to do so, you must first:

✓ Accept the seriousness of the diagnosis.

✓ Regain your emotional balance.

✓ Learn what to avoid and how to avoid it.

✓ Make the necessary changes in your day-to-day activities.

✓ Know what to do in an emergency and be prepared to take charge.

✓ Teach your child how to take charge in your absence.

✓ Teach your child's caregivers and extended community about his condition.

✓ Have faith that you are doing your best and, in so doing, teaching your child to do his best.

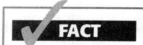

FACT

Less Risky

The death rate from anaphylaxis is very low. In fact, someone who lives with this risk is 10 to 20 times more likely to die in a car accident than from anaphylaxis.

Follow the Basics

Cars are dangerous, but we don't stop our children from riding in them or walking to school. We do, however, ask them to respect the danger, buckle up and follow basic rules. Living safely with allergies is no different.

Taking Precautions

Anaphylactic reactions from food are often preventable. We know that there are usually avoidable mistakes associated with a reaction. They include:

• Failure to check ingredients

• Failure to read a food label

• Delay in administering epinephrine

• Poorly controlled asthma

• An allergy to peanuts, tree nuts or shellfish

• Lack of education about the allergy

Buddy System

◆ ◆ ◆ ◆ ◆

Older children susceptible to exercise-induced anaphylaxis should always exercise with a partner. A buddy can access emergency help should his friend experience a reaction.

Exercise-induced Anaphylaxis

This condition is very rare and not common in children. Symptoms occur during or shortly after physical activity and may range from hives, nausea, vomiting or swelling, to severe difficulties breathing, drop in blood pressure and loss of consciousness. The reaction does not occur with each period of exercise nor with the same amount of exercise.

Certain factors appear to enhance the reaction to exercise:

• Eating any meal less than four hours before exercising

• Eating certain foods like celery, shrimp and wheat

• Taking medications such as aspirin or nonsteroidal anti-inflammatory drugs, such as ibuprofen, before exercising

• Exercising in very hot or cold weather

If you think your child might have exercise-induced anaphylaxis, have him assessed by an allergist.

5 *Key Steps To Take*

1. Notify the school about your child's condition.

2. Make sure your child is supervised during exercise or strenuous play.

3. Ensure he avoids eating up to four hours before exercise.

4. Help your child to avoid the risk factors associated with anaphylaxis (see previous page).

5. Always keep your child's EpiPen on hand.

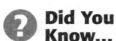 **Did You Know...**

An allergic reaction to an insect sting requires immediate medical attention and can be life threatening if the EpiPen, an injectable medical device containing epinephrine, is not given right away.

LIVING WITH INSECT ALLERGIES

Most children are not allergic to insect stings, but may experience large local reactions. While these reactions can be quite scary, they're not life threatening. A large local reaction occurs when the swelling spreads past the sting site and involves the entire limb or area. The site is very painful, red and swollen, sometimes lasting up to three days. For example, your child could be stung on her foot and a large local reaction can cause her entire leg to swell to twice its size. Your child's doctor may prescribe medications such as antihistamines or corticosteroids to reduce the discomfort if the swelling persists.

Signs and symptoms of an allergic reaction include:

- Hives, swelling and itching on other areas of the body other than the sting site

- Difficulty breathing and chest tightness

- Drooling and coughing in younger children or a hoarse voice

- Vomiting, diarrhea or stomach cramps

- Feeling faint, dizziness or a drop in blood pressure

- Loss of consciousness

Do You Need an Allergist?

If you think that your child has reacted badly to an insect sting, make sure he sees an allergist for an accurate diagnosis. Your allergist will determine his need to carry an EpiPen during insect season and whether he's eligible for desensitization (allergy shots).

10 Tips to Avoid Insects

1. Wear footwear when you're outside; cover up exposed skin when picnicking or camping.

2. Never swat at an insect; if it lands on you, gently brush it away.

3. Don't drink from open beverage cans in the outdoors. Insects often crawl inside.

4. Keep food covered when eating outdoors.

5. Keep garbage away from eating areas.

6. Avoid using perfumes, hair sprays, hair tonics, cosmetics or scented soaps.

7. Don't wear bright or dark clothing. Choose white or tan-colored clothes.

8. Avoid loose clothing or rough fabrics, such as corduroy or denim, in which insects may get trapped.

9. Don't kick at rotting logs or bushes since they can harbor nests.

10. Look for insects before entering a car and keep car windows closed.

Insect Havens

◆ ◆ ◆ ◆ ◆

If your child is at risk of anaphylaxis to insect stings, you should think twice about allowing him to travel to a remote area, such as taking a canoe trip during insect season.

LIVING WITH DRUG ALLERGIES

Allergic reactions to drugs affect a small number of children. The most common cause of allergic reactions is related to antibiotics, particularly penicillin and those drugs in the penicillin family (see *Chapter 8: Drug Allergies*). If your child has been diagnosed with a drug allergy or you suspect that she may have had a reaction, consider the following:

- Have your child assessed by an allergist and skin tested if appropriate.

- Once your allergist confirms a diagnosis, get a MedicAlert identifier for your child.

- Learn the other names of the drugs that your child is also allergic to (for example, penicillin, amoxicillin, cloxacillin).

- Tell other family members and caregivers about your child's drug allergy.

- Ask your allergist to give you a list of medications that you can administer safely to your child.

- Notify your family doctor or pediatrician who cares for your child about his drug allergy, and make sure that it is documented in your child's patient chart.

LIVING WITH LATEX ALLERGY

A latex allergy can vary in severity from mild skin rashes to life-threatening reactions. Unfortunately, it's difficult to predict who will develop more severe symptoms, and who will not. If you suspect your child might be allergic to latex, see an allergist to confirm a diagnosis. Allergy skin testing can be

Drug Relatives

◆ ◆ ◆ ◆ ◆

If your child has a drug allergy, he may also be allergic to a family of drugs. Ask his allergist for the names of those drugs so you can carefully monitor any medication he requires.

done and/or a latex challenge performed (see *Chapter 9: Latex Allergy*).

If your child has had a serious reaction to latex or is at high risk for developing a latex allergy, your allergist may prescribe an EpiPen for your child.

High-risk Groups

- Children with spina bifida or those born with abnormalities in their urinary tracts and require multiple surgeries

- Children with atopy (asthma, rhinitis, eczema)

- Children who have had multiple surgical procedures

- Children with food allergies, particularly to avocado, banana, kiwi or chestnuts

---

ER Alert

♦ ♦ ♦ ♦ ♦

If your child is admitted into a hospital or you go to the emergency department, make sure you tell the nurses and doctors about his latex allergy so that non-latex products may be used during any examination.

The most common source of latex that causes allergic reactions is found in stretchable rubber products, such as balloons, rubber bands, condoms, or the rubber gloves found at your doctor's or dentist's office. Hard rubber products like rubber boots, balls or hard rubber toys are less likely to cause any problems.

If an allergist has confirmed that your child has a latex allergy, make sure you tell your family doctor, pediatrician, and your child's dentist about it so that non-latex gloves and medical supplies are used when your child is examined. Your child should also wear a MedicAlert bracelet or necklace at all times.

Away From Home

Whether your child is traveling or away at camp, take certain precautions to avoid any reactions.

TRAVELING

If you're traveling on an airline, you need to think about the following in advance:

✓ Alert the airline about your child's food allergies, asthma or other health concerns.

✓ Make sure you have extra supplies of medications.

✓ Carry a letter from your doctor, translated into relevant languages, explaining the nature of your child's allergy and the need to carry certain medications.

✓ Some countries (for example, the United States) request that the EpiPen and other injectable medication devices be carried in their original pharmacy packaging.

✓ Have your child wear a MedicAlert bracelet or necklace. This will also help if you have difficulty with security.

✓ Ask your child's allergist if you should be carrying additional medication, such as antihistamines or oral corticosteroids, in case of an emergency.

✓ If your child has a food allergy, check the airlines snack policy.

✓ Make sure that you keep an EpiPen and asthma medication close at hand, and not in an overhead compartment, throughout the trip

✓ If your child has food allergies, do not eat airline food. Risk of cross contact is high, so it's better to just bring your own meals.

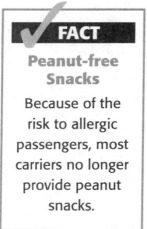

✓ FACT

Peanut-free Snacks

Because of the risk to allergic passengers, most carriers no longer provide peanut snacks.

Before You Travel

- Check on the locations of hospitals or emergency clinics close to where you'll be staying.
- If you're traveling in a foreign country and do not speak the language, have a letter prepared ahead of time outlining your child's condition. Knowing where to get help and preparing for an allergic emergency before it happens will help give you peace of mind while you're traveling.

Be Prepared

◆ ◆ ◆ ◆ ◆

Before you board a plane, contact your local allergy associations for further advice on traveling. They may be able to put you in touch with the allergy association at your destination for further assistance.

AT SCHOOLS, CAMPS AND OTHER CHILD-CARE SETTINGS

Take these steps before enrolling your child.

✓ Ask the principal and teacher about the policies in place at the school/camp.

✓ Provide the necessary information about your child's allergies from your doctor.

✓ Develop an action plan together with your doctor, school/camp and child. Be reasonable with your requests — remember the personnel are generally lay people like yourself and are not medically trained professionals.

✓ Offer to provide training to the staff and students/campers, as well as resource materials available from the various allergy organizations (see the *Resources* section for a full listing of organizations). Most people, even children, are willing to help if they're well informed.

✓ Ensure that when such organizations are planning trips with the children that they are prepared to handle emergencies, are aware of emergency services in the area and can access them easily, for example, with cell phones.

Handling Food

• No trading and sharing of foods, food utensils and food containers should be allowed.

• All food-allergic children should only eat lunches and snacks that have been prepared at home.

• Hand washing is encouraged before and after eating any meal.

• Surfaces such as tabletops, toys, etc., should be washed clean of contaminating foods with soap and water (not just wiped).

• The use of food in crafts and cooking classes may need to be restricted depending on the students' allergies.

• Special training is recommended for school food handlers on what to look for on labels and how to avoid cross contamination.

✔ **FACT**

Inhaling Danger?

The potential risk of life-threatening allergic reactions to airborne food particles, such as peanut butter, is negligible. Therefore, we don't recommend a ban on specific foods based on the risk of reactions from inhaling peanut butter.

Treating an Allergic Reaction

Not all allergic reactions require the use of an EpiPen, a self-injectable device containing epinephrine. For example, reactions to cats are not life threatening; however, reactions to peanut (no matter how mild initially) can be potentially life threatening. If you've received medical advice to carry such a device, follow the instructions on the right.

USING THE EPIPEN: **5** STEPS

1. Pull off the gray safety cap in order to activate the device.

2. Hold the device by placing your hand over the shaft. Don't hold onto either end of the device.

3. Place the black tip firmly against the outer middle part of the thigh *only* and push in until you feel a click. It can be inserted through thin clothing.

4. Hold in place for 10 seconds and then remove it.

5. Call 911. Go by ambulance to the nearest hospital, even if symptoms are mild or have stopped, and properly discard your auto-injector. (The device provides only one injection.)

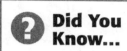 **Did You Know...**

Give epinephrine (EpiPen) at the first sign of a reaction. The first signs may be mild, but symptoms can get worse quickly.

After the EpiPen

After you've administered an EpiPen, remain with your child at all times. Keep her comfortable and calm. Once your child has been rushed to the hospital following an anaphylactic reaction, she'll remain there for three to four hours for observation, even if her symptoms have subsided. The reaction can return. If her symptoms are more severe, then she'll stay for a six- to 12-hour observation period. A life-threatening reaction may require 24-hour observation.

ABOUT THE EPIPEN

✓ Always carry the EpiPen with you, or if your child is comfortable using it, have him carry it at all times.

✓ Keep a record of the expiry date. The EpiPen has an expiry date of 12 to 18 months.

✓ Store at room temperature in its original container/package.

✓ Make sure that the contents are clear, not discolored.

✓ Know how to use it.

✓ Purchase a trainer EpiPen.

✓ Practice with your allergist, clinic nurse or allergy support network.

✓ Teach your child and her caregivers how to use it.

ADMINISTERING THE EPIPEN: 7 COMMON MISTAKES

1. Not having the EpiPen with you when it's needed

2. Not pressing hard enough

3. Injecting the wrong end

4. Holding the thumb over the non-needle end during injection (can interfere with device firing)

5. Handling the black tip

6. Repeating injection unnecessarily

7. Not teaching caregivers how to use it

Double Dose

◆ ◆ ◆ ◆ ◆

Repeat the use of an additional EpiPen in 10 to 15 minutes *only* if the anaphylactic reaction continues or worsens.

Schedule It

◆ ◆ ◆ ◆ ◆

Give your child's caregivers a yearly refresher course on how to use the EpiPen. You'll be surprised at how quickly people forget.

Getting Financial Support

No one should be without an EpiPen for financial reasons. Some allergy associations can assist you with owning one if you're in need. You may also be eligible to receive government support. Check with your allergist or local pharmacist.

Children as Teachers

◆ ◆ ◆ ◆ ◆

Children love to learn new skills. They'll be proud to demonstrate how to work the EpiPen trainer or how to monitor the effectiveness of their asthma medication through the use of a peak flow meter.

Giving our Children the Tools

Our attitude influences our children's attitudes. It's one of the reasons why as a parent you should be an exemplary role model. When we accept the diagnosis of an allergy and demonstrate positive adaptation, we help our child to build what is needed to keep them well, physically and emotionally. We also help them to understand that they're not victims; that allergies create challenges, rather than road blocks. Our children are often more resourceful than we realize. And if we face their growing independence without undue anxiety, it will help them to know that they will be able to handle whatever life throws their way.

It's more important that we teach our children *how* to think rather than *what* to think. While certain rules should be absolute (always carry your EpiPen, etc.), giving children basic principles enables them to think things through for themselves.

DISCUSS THE ALLERGY

When you talk with your child, keep in mind the following:

- Keep it simple, truthful and consistent.

- Choose your words carefully. For example, your child 'lives with the potential for anaphylaxis' but that doesn't make him an 'anaphylactic child.' Teaching your child appropriate language about his allergy will also help him develop a sense of mastery.

- Refuse to make exceptions — this will help your child to feel more secure about his allergy, to take it seriously, and not take chances.

- Role-play with your child. Pretend to be in a restaurant, an airplane, or a school. Encourage her to ask questions and make choices based on the information you give her. Have your child show you what she would do if she thought she was having a reaction, or you were having a reaction.

- From an early age, encourage them to ask questions in restaurants and at school. Give your child opportunities to make decisions.

A Shot at Life

◆ ◆ ◆ ◆ ◆

Some children (and their parents) feel anxious about needles. But if you can accept that a shot of epinephrine could save your child's life, you'll help your child to accept this and to act accordingly. If you feel that you would *not* be able to use the EpiPen, talk with your allergist. She can help you overcome this hurdle.

Finding Role Models

Kids look to role models in everything they do. They'll be encouraged to know, for example, that there are restaurant chefs who work, despite the potential for food-related anaphylaxis, and Olympic athletes who compete, despite their asthma condition. Find out about local, national, international figures who live with similar allergies. It will help your family to keep things in perspective.

Helping Children Live with Allergies

Parents can encourage allergic children to...

Accept the allergy. Encourage allergic children to talk to you, to friends, to schoolmates. It will make it easier for them to accept their allergy as part of who they are when they understand that it does not change the way their peers regard them. You can also help them develop responses to questions or to teasing.

Connect with others who face similar issues. Support groups and monitored websites can help children. Concerns that are left unexplored tend to grow, whereas talking can help put fears into perspective. An older child might enjoy mentoring a younger child — the experience can having a very positive effect on both.

Spin a condition into a positive interest. For example, many children with food allergies love to cook, and there's no reason why this shouldn't be encouraged. Some websites have forums where kids can submit their recipes to share with other children. There are other sites where they can request specific allergen-free recipes. (See the *Resources* section for details.)

Actively manage an allergy. That means children should be encouraged to ask questions in restaurants; to write or call food manufacturers when they have concerns about a product; to make class presentations; to chart their peak flow readings; and to carry their own medications and keep an eye on expiry dates.

Ready and Set

◆ ◆ ◆ ◆ ◆

Your expectations of your child's ability to manage his allergy need to be age-appropriate. No one likes to be singled out. In one case, a father eased his young son's self-consciousness by explaining to servers in restaurants that he and his son both had a food allergy.

Holding On to Hope

Hope, when coupled with realistic expectations, gives us energy to do great things. It enables us to move forward with day-to-day tasks and draw on our creativity to rewrite our story with allergies. Here are some tips to keep you hopeful:

- *Follow the latest developments.* It'll help you feel optimistic about the future, and being part of it will help you feel in charge.

- *Advance advancements.* You or your child might want to participate in research studies, write about advances for a science project or local paper, volunteer with a nonprofit association, start a support group or help raise money.

- *Book regular follow-up visits with your allergist.* Allergies and asthma can change over time and new treatments will become available. The people who maintain the best health are the ones who take an active role in it.

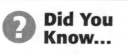 **Did You Know...**

Allergists are specialists in the field of allergic disorders.

Seeking Help

We're sometimes able to find the emotional support that we need through our families, friends and extended community. Often we can gain further benefits by joining a support group or allergy association. Connecting with others who have a similar circumstance can be a powerful way to find relief from our own anxiety. Ask your allergist about resources that could help you and your family. If you or your child is having trouble coping with an allergic condition, you can also explore options for individual or family counseling.

How to Find an Allergist

Allergists are medical doctors who have received specialized training in the field of immunology and allergy. They've received certification in the field by passing examinations supervised by national examining boards. They usually belong to local or national allergy societies that require their members to show proof that they have successfully completed certain exams. These organizations will be able to provide you with the names of qualified allergists in your area (see the *Resources* section for contact information).

National organizations in the United States and Canada that can be contacted include:

- American Academy of Allergy, Asthma & Immunology
- American College of Allergy, Asthma & Immunology
- Canadian Society of Allergy & Clinical Immunology

Dear Diary

◆ ◆ ◆ ◆ ◆

A well-detailed account of your child's activities and health can bring a more accurate diagnosis.

Keeping a Diary

It's important to keep track of when your child's problems get worse so that you may discover what is triggering the problem. Remember, your child will have different triggers as he grows, mainly because of the various exposures he could encounter. Using a diary can help keep track of these occurrences. It can also help your child's allergist make a clearer diagnosis on what is causing his symptoms. Here are some of the questions his allergist might ask:

✓ Where has the child been? School, friend's house, public building, outdoors, etc.? Did the child have to miss school because of her symptoms?

✓ What has the child been around? Animals, tobacco smoke, dusty areas, such as garages, fireplaces, etc.?

✓ What was the weather like during the day? Cold, hot, damp, or was there a rapid change in temperature or humidity?

✓ Has the child been exercising? Running, cycling or even walking? Did these activities have to be stopped?

✓ Does the child have the cold or flu?

✓ Do the problems get worse when she wakes up in the morning or during the night?

✓ Which symptoms is the child experiencing?

THE OUTCOME

Here's just a sampling of some of the factors you'll need to consider when looking for the cause of your child's problems and using a diary. A properly detailed diary can be a great assistant to your child's allergist to help him sort out your child's individual problems.

● *Asthma problems may present in different ways,* such as with recurrent or persistent coughing and/or throat clearing, chest tightness or difficulty breathing. In an asthmatic child, these symptoms may indicate a problem with asthma — wheezing doesn't always have to be present.

Examining Exposures

◆ ◆ ◆ ◆ ◆

Your child may get a reaction to something immediately after exposure or a few hours after coming in contact with a possible allergen. So, if your child is experiencing symptoms, such as a congested nose, cough or wheezing, any possible contact or exposure that occurred earlier must also be examined.

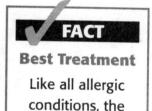
- ***Problems with a runny, stuffy nose*** do not always indicate that your child may have an allergy. This condition is known as rhinitis and allergies are only one possible cause. (See *Chapter 3: Rhinitis* for other possible causes.) Keeping a diary and watching for the effect of nonallergy triggers, such as weather, dry or cold air, perfumes, smoke, etc., is important.

- Similarly, ***looking for the cause of chronic hives*** also can become an exercise in detective work. While most people believe a rash is an allergy and the cause is most likely something that was eaten, the likelihood of that rash being hives and caused by food is very low — about one percent.

  Foods normally produce hives within minutes or within two hours and are gone within one to two days, especially if your child takes an antihistamine. Hives only reappear when that particular food is eaten again. A rash that keeps on reappearing and lasts for several weeks is usually caused by something else. In many of these cases, the cause may never be found.

Finding Answers

Trying to find the cause of your child's problem may not always be easy. Often times, your child will need to see his allergist beyond one visit and undergo allergy skin tests.

Chapter

11

ENVIRONMENTAL CONTROL

Avoiding Allergens and Irritants

ONE OF THE MOST IMPORTANT STEPS IN treating a child's allergies is to avoid the allergen or irritant that causes the illness. This may help decrease the severity of your child's symptoms and reduce the amount of medication she needs for treatment. But first, you'll need to know what allergens cause your child's allergies and then, how to prevent or minimize them daily.

Prevention Lingo

◆ ◆ ◆ ◆ ◆

Avoiding allergens is one way of preventing allergies — also known to the experts as tertiary prevention or the third layer of prevention. See *Chapter 12* for more on primary and secondary prevention.

Avoiding Indoor Allergens

Children who have allergic symptoms all year-round are often allergic to certain things found indoors. This is because they are exposed to these allergens continuously, every day. These allergens include:

- House dust mites
- Indoor molds
- Cockroaches
- Animal dander

HOUSE DUST MITES

These microscopic, spider-like creatures are found in all homes and can cause year-round allergies. Mites live in warm humid places, such as mattresses, pillows, bedding, carpeting and upholstered furniture. It's the mite's dead body parts and feces that create the offending allergens.

Minimize these allergens, particularly in your child's bedroom, with the following measures:

In the bedroom:

✓ Fully encase all pillows (including synthetic non-feather types) and mattresses in specially manufactured, zippered protective coverings to prevent penetration of mites.

✓ Encase box springs with vinyl or plastic.

✓ Use only washable materials on beds. Wash bedding weekly in hot water (55 degrees Celsius/130 degrees Fahrenheit). Dry-cleaning or tumble drying at temperatures greater than 55 degrees Celsius for at least 20 minutes will also kill dust mites.

✓ Remove all dust collectors, such as upholstered furniture, stuffed toys and clutter.

✓ Avoid humidifiers, if possible, in bedrooms since they can collect dust and molds. If humidifying the room is necessary, clean the humidifier daily and ensure it has control dials that will turn the machine off automatically once it's reached a relative humidity of less than 50 percent.

Humidity Hazard

◆ ◆ ◆ ◆ ◆

Humidity greater than 50 percent leads to increased breeding of dust mites.

Chilling/Sizzling Levels

Freezing stuffed toy animals for at least 24 hours has been shown to kill dust mites on their surfaces. However, it will not reduce their allergy properties. Conversely, high temperatures may also affect dust mite levels. For example, exposing carpets to direct sunlight for several hours will kill dust mites, while electric blankets will reduce dust mite growth. However, research shows that none of these methods has any benefits on patients.

Around the house:

✓ Vacuum weekly with a portable or a central vacuum system. There is little evidence that wet vacuum cleaning or steam cleaning is helpful since these practices increase the humidity level in the carpet and foster dust mite growth.

✓ Keep indoor relative humidity between 30 to 50 percent. Humidity levels can be measured with a hygrometer, a device available at most local hardware stores.

✓ Replace carpets with hardwood, linoleum or tile flooring, and keep floors clean.

✓ Replace drapes with washable shades or blinds.

MOLDS OR OTHER FUNGI

Molds are small fungi that grow in areas that are excessively damp, especially where the humidity is more than 50 percent such as in basements, shower stalls, bathroom carpets, air conditioners, humidifiers, vaporizers and on window sills. Some molds or mildew can cause year-round allergic symptoms if they continually reproduce, while other molds are more apparent in certain seasons. Reduce mold exposure with the following measures:

✓ Use an air-conditioning unit in hot weather.

✓ Use a dehumidifier in your home's basement or in a damp area.

✓ Turn on exhaust fans in bathrooms after bathing and in kitchens when cooking.

✓ Install your clothes dryer's vents so they lead to the outside of your home.

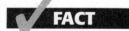

FACT

Fight Mites?

Duct cleaning does not help reduce dust mites, but it may help remove excess dust, debris and, possibly, molds. Air filtration devices are also not very effective for dust control because dust mites do not remain airborne for long periods of time and therefore are not available for filtration.

? Did You Know...

Air filtration devices have been recommended in the past to help remove molds from the air, but researchers have not been able to measure any direct benefit on patients' symptoms.

✓ FACT

Mold Hold

Molds can continually reproduce in damp areas of the house — in this case, they can cause allergic symptoms throughout the year.

✓ Reduce the amount of indoor plants in your living areas.

✓ Don't place carpets directly onto cement basement floors.

✓ Clean washrooms and laundry rooms with five percent bleach solutions.

✓ Clean air conditioners and dehumidifiers frequently.

✓ Clean dust and other debris that have accumulated in air ducts and on furnace filters.

✓ Repair water leaks and areas with water damage.

✓ Avoid living in a damp basement.

✓ Use a dehumidifier in your home's basement or damp areas in order to reduce the amount of humidity, especially if the humidity level is greater than 50 percent.

✓ Avoid using humidifiers and cool or hot mist vaporizers because the mold found in them is difficult to remove. Some of these devices are difficult to regulate and may produce too much humidity or dampness in the room, which is just as much of a problem as is too little humidity or dryness in the room.

COCKROACHES

We now know that the presence of cockroaches is a significant cause of asthma in urban areas. You'll often find cockroaches in inner city dwellings, such as high-rise buildings or schools. They can also be found anywhere in the home, but especially in the kitchen and bedrooms. Here are some ways to eliminate this allergen:

✓ Use pesticides specific for cockroach removal as directed by the manufacturer. These compounds have strange sounding chemical names such as chlorpyrifos, diazanon and boric acid powder.

✓ Hire a professional exterminator. Extermination procedures may also be necessary on adjacent dwellings.

✓ Clean high-traffic areas and food preparation areas, especially the kitchen and eat-ins, regularly, but especially after an extermination procedure.

✓ Repair leaky faucets and pipes. Seal holes in walls and other entry points.

✓ Seal all open food containers and trash cans.

✓ Consider moving to another dwelling, if possible.

HOUSEHOLD ANIMALS

Before making a ruling on whether your household pet is to blame for your child's allergy symptoms, your child should undergo skin testing. A common misconception is that cat and dog allergies are caused by the animals' hair, when in fact they occur because of pet dander (skin scales). Here are some tips on managing pet allergies:

✓ Remove the animal from the home. The benefits may not be apparent until four to six months later because it may take that long to remove animal dander from furnishings, drapes or carpeting in the home.

✓ If pets can't be removed from the home, never allow them into the bedrooms and keep them restricted to one area of the house.

Reel Them In

◆ ◆ ◆ ◆ ◆

Use bait stations containing hydramethylon to control cockroaches. But, remember to keep these products out of the reach of children and pets.

✓ Wash pets once or twice weekly. (Ask the vet for the best method of avoiding skin irritation.) This is a controversial step since animal dander returns within one week of washing so there is only a transient benefit.

✓ Minimize items that trap animal dander, such as carpets and upholstered furniture, and make use of mattress and pillow covers.

✓ Filter the air with a HEPA filter especially in the bedroom — in this case, the HEPA may be helpful because the dander is airborne and will be picked up by the filter.

NOTE: Except for removing a pet from a home, the previous suggestions have not produced consistent clear benefits for the patient. More definitive studies are required in this area.

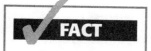

FACT

Pet Pause

There is no such thing as a non-allergenic cat or dog species. Even shorthaired animals can cause allergic symptoms.

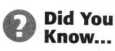

Did You Know...

There are certain times of the day and the year when pollen and mold counts are at their highest. Limit your child's exposure to them by becoming familiar with peak times for pollen and mold growth.

Avoiding Irritants

Like allergens, offending irritants can trigger a child's allergies. Limit their exposure with these tips:

• Avoid tobacco smoke in the home and automobile. (Keep in mind that smoking outdoors still leaves smoke residue on clothing and on one's breath.)

• Control the use of paints, scented products, cleaning agents and perfumes in the home.

• Store chemicals away from the affected individual.

• Use a good ventilation system to remove odors from the home.

Avoiding Outdoor Allergens

It's difficult to avoid pollen and outdoor mold spores altogether, because they are so widespread; however, some control is possible. Start by identifying the pollens your child may be allergic to so you can take extra measures at that time of year.

Pollen/Mold Counts

Here's where and when to expect pollen and mold:

WHAT	WHEN
Tree pollen season	from mid-April to early June in northern and eastern parts of North America
Grass pollen season	from mid-May to the end of July
Ragweed pollen season	from mid-August to October or the first frost
Mold spores	throughout the summer and fall, especially between June and October

Seasonal allergens vary across North America, depending on geographic location. Ask your doctor to help identify specific allergens and seasons in your area.

To reduce your exposure to seasonal allergens: (See *Chapter 3: Rhinitis* for more information.)

✓ Keep windows and doors closed during peak times to prevent the particles from entering the home or car. Use an air conditioner in hot weather to filter out pollen and to lower humidity levels in the home.

✓ When possible, minimize being outside when pollen counts are highest, for example, on sunny and windy days in the morning and afternoon. The counts are lowest immediately after a rainfall, in the evening and at night. (See "Pollen Reports" below for information on pollen forecasts.)

✓ Avoid situations of high exposure to pollen and mold spores, such as when cutting grass, raking leaves, camping, playing in barns and working or near compost heaps.

✓ Don't hang your laundry outside since pollen can collect on clothing.

✓ Very sensitive children may need to wash their hands, face and hair after being outside for long periods of time during the allergy season.

Exposure Limits

◆ ◆ ◆ ◆ ◆

The peak times for exposure to seasonal allergies include: **ragweed** (morning hours); **grass** (afternoon, when it's being mowed); **mold** (after a rainfall, early morning, or when raking leaves).

Pollen Reports

Pollen counts on local weather forecasts aren't often accurate. That's because the level of pollen is usually measured with a sampler placed on the roof of a building. This measure doesn't reflect the pollen count on the street below nor the level a few miles away.

Allergies On The Rise

There have been many studies over time to shed new light on the development of allergies. In this section, we explore some new-age theories in the search for answers on what's causing the increase of allergies in children.

HYGIENE HYPOTHESIS

Recent research shows that asthma, hay fever and eczema seem to be occurring more often as a result of a western lifestyle found in urban industrialized areas. Dubbed the 'hygiene hypothesis,' this concept highlights how better sanitation, less crowded accommodations, better nutrition, more vaccinations and the use of antibiotic medications may have contributed to a decrease in the number of colds and a rise in the amount of allergic diseases, such as asthma, hay fever and eczema, in the general population. There are many questions, however, about the validity of this concept.

For example, cold viruses, such as the RSV (respiratory syncytial virus), can actually bring an increased number of asthma attacks in young children instead of decreasing them as the hygiene hypothesis suggests. Also, whooping cough vaccines have not been shown to lead to a decrease in allergic diseases.

Therefore, until we have more conclusive evidence, we can't put emphasis on this theory, and doctors are not advocating that we get more 'dirty' or stop vaccinating children in order to prevent them from having allergic diseases.

Under Construction

◆ ◆ ◆ ◆ ◆

New theories to uncover the rise of childhood allergies need to be further studied before doctors can use them to diagnose and treat patients.

FARM EXPOSURES

Another hypothesis points to children living in rural or farming communities with having less hay fever and asthma than those who live in urban centers.

The theory is that children living on farms are exposed in the first few years of life to bacteria or a component of the bacteria cell wall known as endotoxin found in stables where animals are housed. However, the research in this area is still inconclusive.

DOMESTIC ANIMAL EXPOSURES

Recent studies show that children who have been exposed to cats and dogs in the early years may actually be protected from developing asthma. This theory contradicts earlier research showing that early animal exposure might actually promote the early development of asthma. But the jury is still out. For example, some research shows that early cat exposures will enhance, instead of reduce, the development of asthma if a child's mother already has asthma. Another study shows that protection is limited only to dogs and not to household cats.

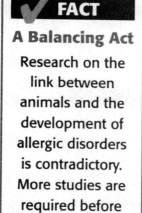

✔ FACT

A Balancing Act

Research on the link between animals and the development of allergic disorders is contradictory. More studies are required before a connection can be made.

The Latest Defense

More recent theories on preventing allergies in children are being investigated. They include altering a mother's diet during pregnancy, breast-feeding protection and introducing solids at a certain age, among other study areas. However, even these are controversial. For more information, see *Chapter 12: Prevention of Allergies.*

PART 4

Looking Forward

Chapter
12

PREVENTION OF ALLERGIES

The Latest Studies on Treating and Avoiding Allergies

THE ABILITY TO PREVENT ALLERGIES HAS BEEN studied for many years and many different approaches have been developed. Research has focused on changes during early infancy since this is the period when the immune system is developing and allergic tendencies usually start to show.

Prevention has been traditionally divided into the following categories:

- **Primary prevention.** Techniques to prevent an allergy from developing.

- **Secondary prevention.** The methods required in preventing further allergies from developing after the allergic disease has appeared in an individual. Many of the techniques for primary prevention are also used at this stage.

- **Tertiary prevention.** Whatever is required to reduce symptoms in patients with both an allergic disorder (for example, asthma, hay fever or eczema) and an associated allergy, such as foods, animal dander, dust mites, molds, pollens (trees, grasses, weeds) that aggravate these disorders.

This chapter focuses on primary and secondary prevention. For a discussion of tertiary prevention, see *Chapter 11: Environmental Control.*

The Latest Research

There have been studies that have tried to modify diet and/or environment to influence the onset of allergies. You should be aware, however, that it's sometimes difficult for your child's physician to advise you one way or another because there are often opposing views from researchers in each of the areas studied in this chapter.

**Researchers
Vs.
Researchers**

◆ ◆ ◆ ◆ ◆

Even with the current body of research available, pediatric associations in North America and Europe don't always agree on their recommendations.

Who Is Studied?

◆ ◆ ◆ ◆ ◆

Recent studies have been conducted on high-risk families where the mother, father and/or a sibling experienced some allergic symptom.

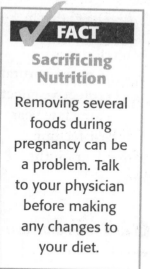

✔ FACT

Sacrificing Nutrition

Removing several foods during pregnancy can be a problem. Talk to your physician before making any changes to your diet.

5 Study Areas

1. Altering a mother's diet during pregnancy

2. Breast-feeding protection

3. Avoiding highly allergenic foods during lactation

4. Modifying the milks used for infant feeding

5. Adding solids to an infant's diet after six months of age

1. MOTHER'S DIET DURING PREGNANCY

There have been studies done during the third trimester of a mother's pregnancy where commonly allergenic foods, such as milk and egg, were either eliminated or given in limited amounts. The mothers also avoided these foods during breast-feeding for the first six months. The children were then followed up to five years of age.

The result: these diets did not appear to have any influence on whether the children developed any allergies. Therefore, altering your diet during pregnancy would have a very minimal effect on the prevention of allergies.

Also, a very restrictive diet may have detrimental effects on the nutrition of the mother and fetus. In fact, elimination diets have been shown to reduce an expectant mother's weight gain by 25 percent, as well as lower the birth weight of the infant.

Eliminating One Food

Some researchers see some benefit in eliminating one food, such as peanut, from a mother's diet, especially if it has a high potential for causing a serious allergy and has little nutritional value. This area is not without opposing views: Some studies have shown that eating peanut during pregnancy did not result in an infant developing a peanut allergy. For parents it's a judgment call — while it may be easier to avoid one food like peanuts instead of several foods to prevent an allergy, this protection may not be perfect.

Research Challenge

♦ ♦ ♦ ♦ ♦

Breast-feeding studies are very difficult to conduct because of the factors that are difficult to control during the infant period. For example, these studies often require large numbers of patients to be on restrictive diets and their environments controlled for months. Conclusions, therefore, are often not clear-cut.

2. BREAST-FEEDING PROTECTION

Many studies in this area have been conducted over the last 60 years to examine whether breast-feeding offers some protection against the development of allergies. To date, however, all the studies that have either shown some benefit or no benefit at all have been riddled with flaws.

But there seems to be some protection from breast-feeding, perhaps because of some of the natural substances found in breast milk. The protective effect is limited. Eczema appears to improve for a few years but not over a lifetime. However, breast-feeding doesn't seem to have any long-term effect on the development of hay fever or asthma.

Recommendations:

According to the American Academy of Pediatrics, current breast-feeding recommendations are:

- Breast-feeding for six months exclusively to offer protection against allergies.

- Breast-feeding should be part of the child's diet until 12 months of age since breast milk has many other benefits, including nutritional, immunological and psychological ones.

3. AVOIDING HIGHLY ALLERGENIC FOODS DURING LACTATION

Nursing mothers have increasingly been interested in what foods to avoid during lactation. It is a fact that trace amounts of milk, egg, wheat and peanut are found in the breast milk of mothers who eat these foods. There is, however, a controversy as to whether this leads to sensitization of the infant to these foods. Some researchers feel this may be happening, but the overall evidence does not support the use of elimination diets.

Recommendations:

The current body of research has resulted in some differing opinions among various medical groups on how nursing moms should structure their diets or whether to include certain foods while nursing.

What mothers need to know is that if they restrict their diets by eliminating certain foods, their child may still develop allergic problems later in life. If you're thinking about eliminating certain foods in your diet, don't forget to seek dietary advice from your doctor before making any restrictions.

These controversies are illustrated by the following different recommendations:

- The American Academy of Pediatrics recommends elimination of peanut and nuts from the diet of the nursing mother (and consideration of milk, egg and fish avoidance). The reason for the recommendation of peanut and nut avoidance is a potential long-term benefit with minimal effect on maternal nutrition. This recommendation is only for those families with a history of allergic disorders.

Nursing Allergies?

◆ ◆ ◆ ◆ ◆

It is controversial whether or not to eliminate highly allergenic foods from the diet of the nursing mother.

- However, the European Society for Paediatric Allergology and Clinical Immunology does not recommend mothers eliminate any specific food during lactation because of the lack of good evidence.

4. MODIFIED MILKS DURING INFANT FEEDING

A) Soy formulas for the treatment of cow's milk allergies.

There's still confusion about the use of soy formulas for the treatment of established cow's-milk allergy. Recent studies show that the incidence of a soy allergy in those with established milk allergies is much lower than once believed.

Recommendation:

Therefore, the Committee on Nutrition of the American Academy of Pediatrics recommends that soy formulas may be used in those infants with a cow's-milk allergy and negative soy oral challenges (see *Chapter 5: Adverse Food Reactions* for more information on oral food challenges). Parents should see benefits within two to four weeks, and the formula continued until the infant is one year of age or older.

Soy Benefits

◆ ◆ ◆ ◆ ◆

According to the Committee on Nutrition of the American Academy of Pediatrics, although soy formulas are not hypoallergenic, they can still be given to some milk-allergic children.

Soy Exceptions

There is one exception to the recommendation above: in the case of rare reactions called *enteropathies*. An infant who experiences this reaction can have severe diarrhea and abdominal upsets when he ingests milk or soy formulas. Since these are not allergic disorders, a skin test to soy or milk may be negative. If milk is identified as the cause of this condition simply by observing a child's reaction following a milk feed, then there's a 60 percent chance that he'll experience a similar problem with a soy formula. In this case, both foods must be avoided.

B) Soy formulas for the prevention of allergies.

The recommendation to use soy formulas for the treatment of soy allergies sometimes confuses people when deciding whether to use such formulas as initial feeds in high-risk families, in order to prevent the development of milk allergies. Several recent studies show that there's no evidence that soy formulas can prevent milk allergies or other allergic conditions, such as eczema and asthma.

Recommendation:

Therefore, The American Academy of Pediatrics, the Australian College of Paediatrics and the Canadian Paediatric Society have all endorsed the policy of *not* recommending soy formulas for the prevention of allergies. The European Society for Paediatric Allergology and Clinical Immunology also agrees with this concept.

> **? Did You Know...**
>
> There is no evidence that soy formula prevents the development of allergic conditions. However, this issue is still being studied.

C) The use of protein hydrolysates in the treatment &/or prevention of atopy.

Formulas that contain casein-based or whey-based hydrolysates have their proteins extensively broken down into smaller amounts to reduce their allergenic properties. In North America, there are three extensively hydrolyzed (broken down) casein preparations. They are:

1. Pregestimil

2. Nutramigen

3. Alimentum

In North America and Europe, a partially hydrolyzed whey formula called Carnation Good Start is available. Profylac, an extensively hydrolyzed whey product, is available in Europe but not in North America.

The more extensively hydrolyzed products may still cause allergic problems but far less than other formulas. For infants who may still have allergic reactions to these formulas, it's recommended they use products that break down proteins even further, to the level of amino acids (which are the backbones of various proteins), such as Neocate for children under one year old and Neocate One for children one year and older.

Recommendations:

1. For the treatment of milk allergies.

Infants with an established cow's milk allergy *and* a documented soy allergy are recommended to use formulas with extensively hydrolyzed casein or extensively hydrolyzed whey. These products may also be used for young infants with cow milk or soy enteropathy. On the other hand, partially hydrolyzed whey formulas, which can trigger a significant number of allergic reactions, should never be used for infants with established cow's-milk allergy.

2. For the prevention of milk and the development of other allergies.

There's some controversy about which preparations are better. Both the extensively and partially hydrolyzed formulas have been associated with preventing the onset of a milk allergy and other allergic disorders up to seven years of age. The

---

Spot the Difference

◆ ◆ ◆ ◆ ◆

Extensively hydrolyzed milk formulas are unlikely to cause allergic reactions in children with cow's-milk protein allergy. However, partially hydrolyzed formulas, such as Carnation Good Start, may still cause some allergic reactions in almost half of milk-allergic children.

extensively hydrolyzed preparations appear to have a slightly better protective effect compared to the partially hydrolyzed preparations. However, like other studies in this field, these studies are difficult to control. More work is required to determine what type of formula is more effective for preventing milk allergy.

- The American Academy of Pediatrics recommends that either extensively hydrolyzed or, in some cases, partially hydrolyzed formula be used.

- The European Society for Paediatric Allergology and Clinical Immunology states that only extensively hydrolyzed formulas be used as a preventive measure.

5. ADDING SOLIDS AFTER SIX MONTHS

Two different studies showed that children who had been exposed to numerous solid foods during the first few months of life had higher rates of eczema in the first few years of life compared to those who didn't start solids until their first year.

Recommendations:

- The American Academy of Pediatrics recommends that solid foods not be introduced until six months of age to children with a high risk of developing allergies. The American group also advises parents about when to add specific foods that have a higher chance of causing allergic reactions into the diet of a child. For example, it suggests the following be added: milk at one year, egg at two years and peanuts, nuts and fish at three years of age.

New Developments

◆ ◆ ◆ ◆ ◆

To learn more about the latest research and recommendations in this area, visit the websites of these organizations (see our *Resources* section on page 238).

- European guidelines do not stress such restrictions, claiming there is not enough evidence for these time frames. They recommend solids be added into an infant's diet after five months of age in any order.

WEIGHING THE RESEARCH

There is no one dietary technique that will prevent allergies (asthma, eczema, hay fever, food allergies) from developing. Avoiding one specific food may modify the development of that specific food allergy, but it has no effect on the development of allergies in general.

Similarly, eczema may be delayed or modified but not completely prevented from developing. There is no effect on the development of hay fever or asthma. While some of these measures may be helpful to some degree, as parents, you need to balance the effort and time to carry out a certain measure without potentially harming your child.

Whatever measure you decide to take, it's important to seek the advice of a medical specialist. Even when recommendations are made — for example, to avoid peanuts until age three — they can never provide 100 percent protection against developing an allergy. When there may be an allergy, in the case of a peanut allergy, your child should be tested and partake in an oral challenge under the supervision of a trained allergist.

Group History

♦ ♦ ♦ ♦ ♦

It's important to note that the suggestions made throughout the chapter are to be used strictly when there is a history of allergies in the family. These measures are not recommended when there is no family history of allergies.

Summary Recommendations

- The use of restrictive diets during pregnancy has been shown to be of little benefit and is not recommended.

- Breast-feeding may be somewhat helpful for preventing allergies. Because of its other health benefits, it's the preferred principal feeding for the first six months of an infant's life, with continued feeding for the rest of the first year.

- The use of restrictive diets during lactation is controversial. The American Academy of Pediatrics recommends nursing mothers avoid highly allergenic foods, such as peanuts, nuts and possibly milk, egg and fish where appropriate. The European Society for Paediatric Allergology and Clinical Immunology does not recommend any specific elimination diet during lactation because of the lack of good evidence.

- Soy milk is not recommended for the prevention of allergies, but may be used to treat established milk allergies.

- Hydrolyzed milk formulas are recommended for the treatment and prevention of milk allergies. Extensively hydrolyzed formulas seem to have a slight advantage over partially hydrolyzed formulas; however, more studies are required.

✔ **FACT**

Seek Professional Advice

Before you decide which course of action to take to change or restrict your child's diet, ask his doctor or allergist for guidance.

GLOSSARY

Acute hives – are the most common form of hives and can appear and disappear spontaneously, lasting minutes, days or weeks (less than six weeks).

Adrenaline (see Epinephrine)

Adverse drug reaction – any noxious, unintended, and undesired effect of a drug that occurs at doses used for prevention, diagnosis, or treatment. It occurs almost 15 out of every 100 times drugs are prescribed by a doctor.

Adverse food reactions – any unwanted reaction after ingesting a food. This includes allergic and nonallergic reactions to food.

Allergic conjunctivitis – an allergic condition of the lining of the eyes causing itchiness, redness and tearing.

Allergic contact dermatitis – a specific immune response with an itchy, red, blistered rash, occurring 24 to 48 hours after contact with an allergen.

Allergic crease – a horizontal crease across the lower part of the nose created by repetitive upward rubbing of the nose.

Allergic march – the term used to describe the progression of different allergies at different ages in children. For example, food allergies and eczema appear in the first two years of life, whereas environmental allergies start to appear in children at ages two or three.

Allergic rhinitis (see Rhinitis)

Allergic shiners – dark bluish discoloration of the lower eyelids caused by nasal congestion.

Allergist – a physician trained as a specialist in the field of allergy/immunology.

Allergy shots/allergy needles (see Immunotherapy)

Ana-Kit – a pre-loaded syringe device that contains two adjustable doses of epinephrine.

Anaphylaxis – a serious allergic reaction that is potentially life threatening. It can occur within minutes or hours of contacting a specific trigger.

Angioedema – swelling of the deeper layers of the skin that can be disfiguring and uncomfortable.

Antihistamines – a group of drugs that block the effects of histamine, one of the natural chemicals the body releases into the tissues and body fluids during an allergic reaction.

Aphids – one of two families from the stinging insects (*hymenoptera*). It includes bumblebees and honeybees.

Applied kinesiology – a controversial test that measures a patient's muscle strength to determine a possible allergy.

Aspartame – a low-calorie sweetener.

Asthma – a disorder that causes the muscles around the bronchial tubes (airways) in the lungs to contract, as well as the lining of the bronchial tubes to become inflamed and swollen.

Asthma anti-inflammatory drugs – a class of medication asthma patients take to help control or eliminate the inflammation so that their airways are less 'twitchy' and asthma symptoms under control. They may be inhaled or swallowed.

Atopic – the genetic tendency to inherit certain allergic disorders such as asthma, hay fever, eczema and food allergy.

Atopic dermatitis (see Eczema)

Bronchodilator – a class of medication that opens the bronchial airways by relaxing the muscles that surround them.

Butylated hydoxyanisole (BHA)/ butylated hydroxytoluene (BHT) – both are antioxidants used in cereals and other grain products to maintain crispiness; they are used in oils to prevent them from going rancid.

Celiac disease – a problem tolerating the gluten found in wheat and other grains. This disease is probably due to an immune response to gluten, but is not an allergic reaction to wheat.

Chronic hives – hives that last more than six weeks. Most of the time, no cause can be identified.

Conjunctivitis (see Allergic conjunctivitis)

Contact dermatitis – a rash caused when the skin comes into contact with irritants or allergens, such as a certain plant or chemical.

Corticosteroids – a class of medications used to decrease inflammation. These medications can be inhaled, topical, injected and oral.

Cytotoxic test – a controversial test where white blood cells (cells used by the body to fight infection) are separated from the rest of the blood and then prepared in a mixture. The cells are then examined at various intervals for any structural changes.

Decongestants – a type of medication that comes in topical and oral forms used to shrink the blood vessels in the nose.

Dermis – a middle layer where the blood vessels, nerves, sweat glands and hair roots are located.

Desensitization – a procedure done where an extremely small amount of an allergen (drug or bee venom) is administered to a patient at increasing doses very slowly until the patient can tolerate the full dose.

Drug allergy – an unpredictable, unexpected adverse reaction to a drug involving IgE antibodies.

Drug interactions – when two or more different drugs are taken together, one may interfere with the action of the other.

Eczema *(also known as atopic dermatitis)* – a common chronic skin disease that causes itchy, red, raised and scaly skin. It is often associated with other allergies.

Electrodermal Testing *(also known as vega test)* – a controversial test that uses a galvanometer to measure electrical activity of the skin at specific acupuncture points.

Elimination diet – a diet that involves eliminating a suspect allergenic food, usually done for one to two weeks.

Enteropathies – gastrointestinal reactions that have no connection to allergies, but may occur from milk, soy and other food in the diet.

Eosinophil – a specialized white blood cell that may increase in number in allergic children.

Epidermis – the skin's outer protective layer.

Epinephrine *(also known as adrenaline)* – a hormone produced by the body's adrenal glands in response to stressful situations. In drug form, it is the first line of medication used to treat anaphylaxis.

EpiPen – an auto-injectable device with epinephrine, which is available in two doses.

Eye allergies (see Allergic conjunctivitis)

Food allergy – an allergic disorder that typically occurs immediately or soon after eating a specific food. In this case, the immune system responds adversely to a food protein that is usually tolerated by nonallergic individuals.

Food diary – a record of all the foods eaten at each meal, how the foods were prepared and the nature and times of the onset of symptoms.

Food intolerance – an adverse reaction to a food that is nonallergic.

Food-pollen allergy syndrome *(also known as oral allergy syndrome and fresh-fruit syndrome)* – an allergic reaction to certain proteins in a variety of fresh fruits, raw vegetables and nuts and seeds, which develops in some people with pollen allergies.

Fresh-fruit syndrome (see Food-pollen allergy syndrome)

Generalized allergic reaction – an allergic reaction that usually involves areas of the body — most often the skin, throat, lungs, heart and digestive system.

Hay fever (see Seasonal allergic rhinitis)

Hives *(also known as urticaria)* – welts on the skin that can vary in shape and color, and last for hours, days, weeks, months or years.

Hydrolyzed baby formulas – a type of infant formula that has its proteins broken down (hydrolyzed) into smaller units.

Hymenoptera – stinging insects made up of two families, aphids and vespids.

Hypoallergenic – less allergenic.

Hyposensitization (see Immunotherapy)

ImmunoCap blood test – a newer version of the RAST used to help determine if a patient has IgE antibodies to specific allergens.

Immunoglobulin E (IgE) antibodies – various proteins produced by the immune system that are specifically associated with allergies.

Immunotherapy *(also known as allergy shots, desensitization or hyposensitization)* – a preventive treatment for allergy to pollens (trees, grasses, weeds), house dust mites, molds and insect stings.

Irritant contact dermatitis – a type of skin rash characterized with redness, dryness, cracking, scaling and blisters secondary to an irritant such as soap and detergent. This is not an allergic reaction.

Irritants – substances that directly harm the body without involving an allergic response. For example, cold air, tobacco smoke and paint fumes may affect the lungs while soap and detergents may affect the skin.

Lactase – an enzyme that helps digest or break down the sugar in milk (lactose) and certain milk products.

Lactose – the predominant sugar in milk and certain milk products.

Lactose intolerance – the inability to digest lactose, the main sugar found in milk and dairy products. This is NOT a food allergy.

Latex *(also known as natural rubber latex)* – a substance that comes from the sap of the rubber tree (*Hevea brasiliensis*) found primarily in Africa and Southeast Asia, and is commonly used to make medical supplies, household products and toys.

Local anaesthetics – a group of medications used to decrease the pain involved during dental procedures and other minor procedures.

Localized reaction *(to insect stings)* – a response that involves redness and swelling at the involved site and may affect adjacent areas.

MMR vaccine – a vaccination that protects against measles, mumps and rubella.

Malabsorption syndromes – conditions that interfere with the absorption of foods.

Monosodium glutamate (MSG) – a food additive used to enhance flavor.

Natural rubber latex (see Latex)

Neoprene – a latex alternative used to make products such as gloves.

Nitrates and nitrites – curing agents used in meat products, for example, salami, ham and bologna.

Nonallergic rhinitis – inflammation in the nose caused by viral infections and irritants such as cigarette smoke, perfumes, paint smells, and extremes of cold, hot or damp weather.

Non-steroidal anti-inflammatory drugs (NSAIDs) – drugs used to treat pain, fever and joint inflammation.

Oral corticosteroids (see Corticosteroids)

Oral allergy syndrome (see Food-pollen allergy syndrome)

Oral food challenge – the most reliable test for confirming a true food allergy. The test involves feeding a child increasing amounts of a suspect food. If there is the potential for a severe reaction, this is always done under a doctor's supervision where treatment can be given immediately if there is a serious reaction.

Peak flow meter – a device used to monitor how well your child's asthma is controlled.

Perennial allergic rhinitis – an allergic condition with symptoms such as sneezing, clear watery discharge and a congested nose that occur throughout the year. It is caused by indoor allergens, such as house dust mite, animal dander, indoor molds and cockroaches.

Phototherapy – a treatment using ultra-violet light waves to treat severe eczema.

Primary prevention – techniques to prevent an allergy from developing.

Provocation-neutralization – a controversial test that aims to expose the patient to doses of various allergens intradermally (into the skin), subcutaneously (under the skin), or sublingually (under the tongue) to treat their allergies.

Provocative drug testing – a procedure conducted when a patient must take a specific medication, for which there is no skin test available, to determine whether or not they will have an adverse reaction.

Radioallergosorbent test (RAST) – a blood test that measures the level of a specific antibody called IgE, which the body produces in response to specific antigens like ragweed or grass pollen. It's used when skin testing is not an option.

Rhinitis – inflammation (redness and swelling) of the lining of the nose.

Rhinitis medicamentosa – a chronic stuffy nose from prolonged use of over-the-counter decongestant nasal sprays.

Seasonal allergic rhinitis (also known as hay fever) – an allergic condition where an individual experiences symptoms at certain times of the year, like spring, summer or fall. Pollens (trees, grasses or weeds) or outdoor molds are the prime culprits.

Secondary prevention – methods required in preventing further allergies from developing after the allergic disease has appeared in an individual.

Signs (see Symptoms) – what doctor finds when examining the patient, for example, facial swelling, hives or wheezing.

Skin prick test – a common allergy test done by placing drops of allergen extracts on the back or forearm and then lightly pricking the skin. The skin test should always be interpreted together with the patient's history.

Sodium benzoate/benzoic acid – both are used widely to inhibit the growth of microorganisms in foods such as cereals, cakes and instant potatoes. Benzoic acid also occurs naturally in cranberries, raspberries, prunes and other foods.

Soy-based formulas – a type of infant formula that uses the proteins from soybeans rather than those found in cow's milk.

Sulfite – a type of preservative used to prevent foods from browning and spoiling.

Symptoms (see Signs) – what the patient tells the physician they are experiencing, such as itching, dizziness or shortness of breath.

Tar ointments – a treatment used very rarely to soothe inflamed skin.

Tartrazine – a synthetic food coloring agent (yellow dye #5) found in cake and icing mixes, puddings, pie fillings, ice creams, drink mixes and soft drinks.

Tertiary prevention – whatever is required to reduce symptoms in patients who have already been diagnosed with an allergic condition, such as allergic rhinitis, asthma and eczema.

Topical corticosteroids (see Corticosteroids)

Type-1 allergic reaction – an immune response that involves the production of the specific Immunoglobulin E (IgE) antibody.

Urticaria (see Hives)

Vasomotor rhinitis – a form of rhinitis that is neither allergic nor infectious. It develops from an imbalance of the systems that regulate the nose lining, including the nerves and blood vessels within the nose.

Vega test (see Electrodermal testing)

Vespids – one of two families from the *hymenoptera* (stinging insects). It includes the yellow jacket, yellow hornet, white-faced hornet and wasp.

Wheezing – a particular whistling sound caused by constriction of the bronchial tubes.

Year-round allergies (see Perennial allergic rhinitis)

RESOURCES

For more information on allergic disorders, contact the following organizations. Many of these organizations have links to other sites that you may find useful.

FOR GENERAL ALLERGIES

American Academy of Allergy, Asthma & Immunology

611 East Wells St.
Milwaukee, WI 53202
Tel.: (414) 272-6071
Patient Information and Physician Referral Line:
(800) 822-2762
www.aaaai.org
E-mail: info@aaaai.org

The AAAAI has more than 6,000 members practicing as allergist/immunologists and allied health professionals dedicated to advancing the knowledge and practice of allergic disease and the Academy's mission of optimal patient care.

American College of Allergy, Asthma & Immunology

85 West Algonquin Rd., Suite 550
Arlington Heights, IL 60005
Tel.: (847) 427-1200
Fax: (847) 427-1294
www.acaai.org
Public education site: http://allergy.mcg.edu/

The ACAAI is a professional association of 4,000 allergists/immunologists dedicated to improving the quality of patient care in allergy and immunology through research, advocacy and professional and public education.

Canadian Society of Allergy & Clinical Immunology (CSACI)

774 Echo Dr.
Ottawa, ON K1S 5N8
Tel.: (613) 730-6272
Fax: (613) 730-1116
www.csaci.medical.org
E-mail: csaci@rcpsc.edu

The CSACI, among other goals, strives to improve the standards of teaching and practice of allergy and clinical immunology, as well as foster cooperation between those engaged in the study and practice of allergy and clinical immunology.

European Academy of Allergology and Clinical Immunology (EAACI)

Executive Office Sweden, Executive Manager C. OSTROM
Box 24140
S-104 51 Stockholm, Sweden
www.eaaci.net/site/homepage.php
E-mail: executive.office@eaaci.org

The EAACI is an association including 39 European national societies, more than 3,500 academicians, research investigators and clinicians aimed at promoting basic and clinical research, as well as collecting, assessing and disseminating scientific information.

American Academy of Pediatrics

141 Northwest Point Blvd.
Elk Grove Village, IL 60007-1098
Tel.: (847) 434-4000
Fax: (847) 434-8000
www.aap.org/
E-mail: kidsdocs@aap.org

The American Academy of Pediatrics and its member pediatricians dedicate their efforts and resources to the health, safety and well-being of all infants, children, adolescents and young adults. It has references about allergies on its website and information about research being done on the prevention of allergies.

Allergy/Asthma Information Association (AAIA)

Box 100
Toronto, ON M9W 5K9
Tel.: (416) 679-9521 or (800) 611-7011 (Toll free)
Fax: (416) 679-9524
www.calgaryallergy.ca/aaia/aboutaaia.htm
E-mail: national@aaia.ca

The AAIA is a support group that offers resources to help individuals find the most effective ways to tackle their allergy and asthma problems. It was founded as a voluntary organization in 1964 by concerned parents of allergic children who set out to get labelling on food.

The Hospital for Sick Children

Division of Immunology/Allergy

555 University Ave.
Toronto, ON M5G 1X8
Tel.: (416) 813-1500
Website under construction at time of printing.

The Hospital for Sick Children is a world-renowned health-care, teaching and research center dedicated exclusively to children; affiliated with the University of Toronto. The division of Immunology/Allergy at The Hospital for Sick Children is involved in research, teaching and care of patients with immunological and allergic disorders.

FOR SPECIFIC ALLERGIES

Asthma:

Asthma Society of Canada

130 Bridgeland Ave., Suite 425
Toronto, ON M6A 1Z4
Tel.: (416) 787-4050 or (800) 787-3880 (Toll Free)
Fax: (416) 787-5807
www.asthmasociety.com
www.asthmakids.ca

The Asthma Society is the only national registered charity that focuses on asthma education and research.

American Lung Association

(childhood asthma site)
61 Broadway, 6th Floor
NY, NY 10006
Tel.: (212) 315-8700 or (800) LUNG-USA (800-586-4872)
www.lungusa.org/asthma/

The American Lung Association is the oldest voluntary health organization in the United States. Today, it fights lung disease in all its forms, with special emphasis on asthma, tobacco control and environmental health.

Canadian Lung Association (asthma)

3 Raymond St., Suite 300
Ottawa, ON K1R 1A3
Tel.: (613) 569-6411
Fax: (613) 569-8860
www.lung.ca/asthma/index.html
E-mail: info@lung.ca

The Lung Association is nonprofit and volunteer-based organization whose chief purpose is to combat both disease and environmental threats to the lungs.

Eczema:

American Academy of Dermatology (AAD)

1350 I St. NW, Suite 880
Washington, DC 20005-4355
Tel.: (202) 842-3555
Fax: (202) 842-4355
www.aad.org
E-mail (Communications Department): yurbikas@aad.org

The American Academy of Dermatology is the largest and most representative of all dermatologic associations. The site has a wealth of information on allergic skin diseases.

National Eczema Association for Science and Education (NEASE)

4460 Redwood Hwy., Ste. 16-D
San Rafael, CA 94903-1953
Tel.: (415) 499-3474 or (800) 818-7546 (Toll Free)
Fax: (415) 472-5345
www.nationaleczema.org
E-mail: info@nationaleczema.org

NEASE works to improve the health and the quality of life of persons living with atopic dermatitis/eczema, including those who have the disease as well as their loved ones.

Food:

Canadian Food Inspection Agency

Website for allergy alerts
http://www.inspection.gc.ca/english/toce.shtml

The Canadian Food Inspection Agency delivers all federal inspection services related to food, animal health and plant protection.

Food and Drug Administration

5600 Fishers Lane
Rockville, Maryland 20857
Tel.: (888) INFO-FDA (888-463-6332)
www.fda.gov

The FDA, among other responsibilities, promotes public health by promptly and efficiently reviewing clinical research and taking appropriate action on the marketing of regulated products in a timely manner.

The Food Allergy & Anaphylaxis Network

10400 Eaton Pl., Suite 107
Fairfax, VA 22030-2208
Tel.: (800) 929-4040
www.foodallergy.org
E-mail: faan@foodallergy.org

FAAN helps to raise public awareness, to provide advocacy and education, and to advance research on behalf of all those affected by food allergies and anaphylaxis. The site also provides allergy-free recipes.

Specialty Food Shop at The Hospital for Sick Children

The Hospital for Sick Children (Main Floor, Concourse)
555 University Ave.
Toronto, ON M5G 1X8
Tel: (416) 977-4360 or (800) 737-7976 (Toll free)
Fax: (416) 977 8394
www.specialtyfoodshop.com
E-mail: sfs@sickkids.ca

The Speciality Food Shop provides specialized nutritional products for people of any age with any health concern. Owned and operated by The Hospital for Sick Children.

Anaphylaxis:

Anaphylaxis Canada

416 Moore Ave., Suite 306
Toronto, ON M4G 1C9
Tel.: (416) 785-5666
Fax: (416) 785-0458
www.anaphylaxis.org
Children's website: www.safe4kids.ca
E-mail: info@anaphylaxis.ca

Anaphylaxis Canada is a nonprofit organization created by and for people with anaphylaxis. Among other services, it provides information and support to people with anaphylaxis and works to improve safety standards for people with anaphylaxis.

MedicAlert Foundation International

2323 Colorado Ave.
Turlock, CA 95382
Tel.: (209) 668-3333 or (888) 633-4298 (Toll free)
www.medicalert.com

MedicAlert is the leading provider of medical information services that are linked to customized medical bracelets and necklets (necklaces).

Latex:

A.L.E.R.T. (Allergy to Latex Education and Resource Team)

American Latex Allergy Association
3791 Sherman Rd.
Slinger, WI 53086
Tel.: (888) 972-5378 (Toll Free)
Fax: (262) 677-2808
www.latexallergyresources.org
E-mail: alert@execpc.com

A.L.E.R.T. is a national nonprofit, tax exempt organization that has designed this website to help connect you with educational materials, support groups, publications and product information to assist you with your understanding of natural rubber latex allergy.

National Institute for Occupational Safety and Health (NIOSH)

4676 Columbia Parkway
Cincinnati, OH 45226-1998
Tel.: (800) 35-NIOSH (800-356-4674)
Fax: (513) 533-8573
www.cdc.gov/niosh/homepage.html
Latex: www.cdc.gov/niosh/latexalt.html
E-mail: pubstaft@cdc.gov

NIOSH is the federal agency responsible for conducting research and making recommendations for the prevention of work-related disease and injury. The Institute is part of the Centers for Disease Control and Prevention.

Occupational Safety & Health Administration (OSHA)

U.S. Department of Labor
200 Constitution Ave.
Washington, D.C. 20210
Tel.: (800) 321-OSHA (6742) (Toll Free U.S.)
www.osha.gov
Latex Allergy: www.osha.gov/SLTC/latexallergy/index.html

OSHA's mission is to ensure safe and healthful workplaces in America.

Spina Bifida Association Of America

4590 MacArthur Blvd., NW, Suite 250
Washington, DC 20007-4226
Tel.: (202) 944-3285 or (800) 621-3141 (Toll Free)
Fax: (202) 944-3295
www.sbaa.org (see Latex Issues)
E-mail: sbaa@sbaa.org

Spina Bifida Association of America promotes the prevention of spina bifida and enhances the lives of all affected.

Pediatrics:

Canadian Paediatric Society (CPS)

100-2204 Walkley Rd.
Ottawa ON K1G 4G8
Tel.: (613) 526-9397
Fax: (613) 526-3332
www.cps.ca
E-mail: info@cps.ca

The CPS has more than 2,000 paediatrician members from across Canada and several hundred volunteers as members. These experts are responsible for creating or reviewing all the educational materials it produces for parents. The CPS is also involved in the education of pediatricians, family physicians and others who care for children.

INDEX